SEIDEL'S
PHYSICAL EXAMINATION
HANDBOOK: AN INTERPROFESSIONAL APPROACH NINTH EDITION

JANE W. BALL, RN, DRPH, CPNP
Trauma Systems Consultant, American College of Surgeons, Gaithersburg, Maryland

JOYCE E. DAINS, DRPH, JD, RN, FNP-BC, FNAP, FAANP
Professor and Director Advanced Practice Nursing, The University of Texas, M. D. Anderson Cancer Center, Houston, Texas

JOHN A. FLYNN, MD, MBA, MED
Clinical Director and Professor of Medicine, Division of General Internal Medicine, The Johns Hopkins University, School of Medicine, Baltimore, Maryland

BARRY S. SOLOMON, MD, MPH
Associate Professor of Pediatrics, Assistant Dean for Student Affairs, Division of General Pediatrics and Adolescent Medicine, The Johns Hopkins University, School of Medicine, Baltimore, Maryland

ROSALYN W. STEWART, MD, MS, MBA
Associate Professor of Pediatrics and Medicine, Department of Internal Medicine and Pediatrics, The Johns Hopkins University, School of Medicine, Baltimore, Maryland

ELSEVIER

ELSEVIER

3251 Riverport Lane
St. Louis, Missouri 63043

SEIDEL'S PHYSICAL EXAMINATION
HANDBOOK, NINTH EDITION

ISBN: 978-0-323-54532-7

Notices

Knowledge and best practice in this field are constantly changing. As new research and experience broaden our understanding, changes in research methods, professional practices, or medical treatment may become necessary.

Practitioners and researchers must always rely on their own experience and knowledge in evaluating and using any information, methods, compounds, or experiments described herein. In using such information or methods, they should be mindful of their own safety and the safety of others, including parties for whom they have a professional responsibility.

With respect to any drug or pharmaceutical products identified, readers are advised to check the most current information provided (i) on procedures featured or (ii) by the manufacturer of each product to be administered and to verify the recommended dose or formula, the method and duration of administration, and contraindications. It is the responsibility of practitioners, relying on their own experience and knowledge of their patients, to make diagnoses, to determine dosages and the best treatment for each individual patient, and to take all appropriate safety precautions.

To the fullest extent of the law, neither the Publisher nor the authors, contributors, or editors assume any liability for any injury and/or damage to persons or property as a matter of products liability, negligence or otherwise, or from any use or operation of any methods, products, instructions, or ideas contained in the material herein.

Executive Content Strategist: Lee Henderson
Content Development Manager: Luke Held
Content Development Specialist: Kelly Skelton
Publishing Services Manager: Deepthi Unni
Project Manager: Apoorva V
Design Direction: Muthukumaran Thangaraj

Working together
to grow libraries in
developing countries

www.elsevier.com • www.bookaid.org

Printed in China

Last digit is the print number: 9   8   7   6   5   4   3   2   1

Preface

Seidel's Physical Examination Handbook: An Interprofessional Approach, ninth edition, is a portable clinical reference on physical examination that is suitable for students of nursing, medicine, chiropractic, osteopathic, and other allied health disciplines, as well as for practicing health care providers. It offers brief descriptions of examination techniques and guidelines on how the examination should proceed, step by step. This handbook is intended to be an aid to review and recall the procedures of physical examination. Because of its brevity, specific techniques of history taking by organ system are not described.

The handbook begins with an outline of what information should be obtained for the patient's medical history and review of systems. Subsequent chapters for each of the body systems list equipment needed to perform the examination and present the techniques to be used. Expected and Unexpected Findings follow the description of each technique, presented in distinctive color type for easy recognition. Numerous illustrations interspersed throughout the text reinforce techniques and possible findings. Pediatric examination variations are highlighted in each body systems chapter.

Each chapter offers Aids to Differential Diagnosis and also provides Sample Documentation, which is focused on a specific patient concern to illustrate good documentation practice. Subjective Data and Objective Data are clearly differentiated for each abnormality in the Aids to Differential Diagnosis section of each chapter in the ninth edition.

As in previous editions, separate chapters give an overview of the entire examination for all adults; for infants, children, and adolescents; for older adults; and for healthy female patients. The final chapter gives guidelines for documentation findings.

Jane W. Ball
Joyce E. Dains
John A. Flynn
Barry S. Solomon
Rosalyn W. Stewart

To Henry W. Seidel and
G. William Benedict

We dedicate the ninth edition of this text to the two original authors, Henry M. Seidel, MD, and William Benedict, MD. Both physicians had academic appointments at the Johns Hopkins University School of Medicine for decades and made important contributions to patient care and medical student education in their specialties of pediatrics and endocrinology/internal medicine, respectively.

As original authors, they contributed greatly to the initial text design as well as to its ongoing development. Both Dr. Seidel and Dr. Benedict understood the importance of communication, sensitivity, compassion, and connection with patients. This text was one of the earliest collaborations of a physician and nurse author team, in this case to develop a text targeted to students of medicine, nursing, and other allied health professions. The ability of these physicians to merge their visions with that of the nurse authors and to collaborate as an effective team allowed the authors to shape this text and share important values with students.

The History

Building the History

The following outline of a patient history is a guideline and should not be considered a rigid structure. You are beginning your relationship with the patient at this point. Choose a comfortable setting, and help the patient get settled. Maintain eye contact, and use a conversational tone. Begin by introducing yourself and explaining your role. Help the patient understand why you are building the history and how it will be used. Use open-ended questions to begin and explore responses with additional questions: where, when, what, how, and why. Be sensitive to the patient's emotions. Avoid confrontation and leading questions.

Chief Concern

* Problem or symptom: reason for visit
* Duration of problem
* Other concerns: secondary issues, fears, concerns, what made patient seek care
* Always consider why this particular problem may be affecting this particular patient at this time. Why did this patient succumb to a risk or an exposure when others similarly exposed did not?

History of Present Illness

When more than one problem is identified, address each problem separately.
* Chronologic ordering: sequence of events patient has experienced
* State of health just before onset of present problem
* Complete description of first symptom: time and date of onset, location, movement
* Possible exposure to infection or toxic agents
* If symptoms are intermittent, describe typical episode: onset, duration, symptoms, variations, inciting factors, exacerbating factors, relieving factors
* Effect of illness on: lifestyle, ability to function; limitations imposed by illness
* "Stability" of problem: intensity, variations, improvement, worsening, staying the same

- Reason for seeking attention, particularly for long-standing problem
- Review of affected system when there is a disturbance of a particular organ or system
- Medications tried: current and recent, dosage of prescriptions, nonprescription medications
- Use of complementary or alternative therapies and medications; home remedies
- At conclusion, review of chronology of events for each problem: patient's confirmations and corrections

Medical History

- Hospitalizations and/or surgeries (including outpatient surgeries): dates, hospital, diagnosis, complications, injuries, disabilities
- Childhood illnesses: measles, mumps, pertussis, varicella, scarlet fever, rheumatic fever
- Adult illnesses: tuberculosis, hepatitis, diabetes mellitus, hypertension, coronary artery disease/myocardial infarction, tropical or parasitic infection, other infections
- Serious injuries: traumatic brain injury, liver laceration, spinal injury, fractures
- Immunizations: polio, diphtheria, pertussis, tetanus toxoid, hepatitis B, measles, mumps, rubella, *Haemophilus influenzae,* varicella, influenza, hepatitis A, meningococcal, human papillomavirus, pneumococcal, zoster, typhoid, anthrax, smallpox, bacille Calmette-Guérin, last tuberculin skin test, unusual reaction to immunizations
- Medications: past, current, and recent medications (dosage, nonprescription medications, vitamins); complementary and herbal therapies
- Allergies: drugs, foods, environmental allergens along with the allergic reaction (e.g., rash, anaphylaxis)
- Transfusions: reason, date, and number of units transfused; reaction, if any
- Mental health: mood disorders, psychiatric therapy or medications
- Recent laboratory tests: glucose, cholesterol, Pap smear/human papillomavirus (HPV), HIV, mammogram, colonoscopy or fecal occult blood test, prostate-specific antigen

Family History

The genetic basis for a patient's response to risk or exposure may determine whether the patient becomes ill when others do not.

- Relatives with similar illness
- Immediate family: ethnicity, health, cause of and age at death

- History of disease: heart disease, high blood pressure, hypercholesterolemia, cancer, tuberculosis, stroke, epilepsy, diabetes, gout, kidney disease, thyroid disease, asthma and other allergic states, forms of arthritis, blood diseases, sexually transmitted infections, other familial diseases
- Spouse and children: age, health
- Hereditary disease: history of grandparents, aunts, uncles, siblings, cousins; consanguinity

Personal and Social History

- Cultural background and practices, birthplace, where raised, home environment as youth, education, position in family, marital status, gender identity and sexual orientation, general life satisfaction, hobbies, interests, sources of stress, religious preference (religious or cultural proscriptions concerning medical care)
- Home environment: number of individuals in household, pets, economic situation
- Occupation: usual work and present work if different, list of job changes, work conditions and hours, physical or mental strain, duration of employment; present and past exposure to heat and cold, industrial toxins; protective devices required or used; military service
- Environment: home, school, work, structural barriers if physically disabled, community services utilized; travel and other exposure to contagious diseases, residence in tropics; water and milk supply, other sources of infection when applicable
- Current health habits and/or risk factors: exercise; smoking (pack years: packs per day × duration); salt intake; obesity/weight control; diet; alcohol intake: (amount/day), duration; CAGE (Cutting down, Annoyance by criticism, Guilty feeling, Eye-openers) or TACE (Take, Annoyed, Cut down, Eye-opener) question responses (see Appendix on special histories); recreational drugs and methods (e.g., injection, ingestion, sniffing, smoking, or use of shared needles)
- Exposure to chemicals, toxins, poisons, asbestos, or radioactive material at home or work and duration; caffeine use (cups/glasses/day)
- Sexual activity: contraceptive or barrier protection method used; past sexually transmitted infections; treatment
- Screen for intimate partner violence: see Appendix on special histories
- Complementary and alternative health and medical systems: history and current use

THE HISTORY

- Religious preference: religious proscriptions concerning medical care
- Concerns about cost of care, health care coverage

Review of Systems

It is unlikely that all questions in each system will be asked on every occasion. The following questions are among those that should be asked, particularly at the first interview:

- General constitutional symptoms: fever, chills, malaise, easily fatigued, night sweats, weight (average, preferred, present, change over a specified period and whether this change was intentional)
- Skin, hair, and nails: rash or eruption, itching, pigmentation or texture change; excessive sweating, unusual nail or hair growth
- Head and neck: frequent or unusual headaches, their location, dizziness, syncope; brain injuries, concussions, loss of consciousness (momentary or prolonged)
- Eyes: visual acuity, blurring, double vision, light sensitivity, pain, change in appearance or vision; use of glasses/contacts, eye drops, other medication; history of trauma, glaucoma, familial eye disease
- Ears: hearing loss, pain, discharge, tinnitus, vertigo
- Nose: sense of smell, frequency of colds, obstruction, nosebleeds, postnasal discharge, sinus pain
- Throat and mouth: hoarseness or change in voice; frequent sore throats, bleeding or swelling of gums; recent tooth abscesses or extraction; soreness of tongue or buccal mucosa, ulcers; disturbance of taste
- Lymphatic: enlargement, tenderness, suppuration
- Chest and lungs: pain related to respiration, dyspnea, cyanosis, wheezing, cough, sputum (frequency, character, and quantity), hemoptysis, night sweats, exposure to tuberculosis; last chest radiograph
- Breasts: development, pain, tenderness, discharge, lumps, galactorrhea, mammograms (screening or diagnostic), breast biopsies
- Heart and blood vessels: chest pain or distress, precipitating causes, timing and duration, relieving factors, palpitations, dyspnea, orthopnea (number of pillows), edema, hypertension, previous myocardial infarction, exercise tolerance (flights of steps, distance walking), past electrocardiogram and cardiac tests
- Peripheral vasculature: claudication (frequency, severity), tendency to bruise or bleed, thromboses, thrombophlebitis

- Hematologic: anemia, any known blood cell disorder
- Gastrointestinal: appetite, digestion, intolerance of any foods, dysphagia, heartburn, nausea, vomiting, hematemesis, bowel regularity, constipation, diarrhea, change in stool color or contents (clay, tarry, fresh blood, mucus, undigested food), flatulence, hemorrhoids, hepatitis, jaundice, dark urine; history of ulcer, gallstones, polyps, tumor; previous radiographic studies, sigmoidoscopy, colonoscopy (where, when, findings)
- Diet: appetite, likes and dislikes, restrictions (because of religion, allergy, or other disease), vitamins and other supplements, caffeine-containing beverages (coffee, tea, cola); food diary or daily listing of food and liquid intake as needed
- Endocrine: thyroid enlargement or tenderness, heat or cold intolerance, unexplained weight change, polydipsia, polyuria, changes in facial or body hair, increased hat and glove size, skin striae
  - Male patients: puberty onset, erections, emissions, testicular pain, libido, infertility
  - Female patients: menses onset, regularity, duration, amount of flow; dysmenorrhea; last period; intermenstrual discharge or bleeding; itching; date of last Pap smear/HPV test; age at menopause; libido; frequency of intercourse; sexual difficulties
- Pregnancy: infertility; gravidity and parity (G = number of pregnancies, P = number of childbirths, A = number of abortions/miscarriages, L = number of living children); number and duration of each pregnancy, delivery method; complications during any pregnancy or postpartum period; use of oral or other contraceptives
- Genitourinary: dysuria, flank or suprapubic pain, urgency, frequency, nocturia, hematuria, polyuria, hesitancy, dribbling, loss in force of stream, passage of stone; edema of face, stress incontinence, hernias, sexually transmitted infection
- Musculoskeletal: joint stiffness, pain, restriction of motion, swelling, redness, heat, bony deformity, number and pattern of joint involvement
- Neurologic: syncope, seizures, weakness or paralysis, problems with sensation or coordination, tremors
- Mental health: depression, mania, mood changes, difficulty concentrating, nervousness, tension, suicidal thoughts, irritability, sleep disturbances

THE HISTORY

Concluding Questions

- Is there anything else that you think would be important for me to know?
- If there are several problems: Which concerns you the most?
- If the history is vague, complicated, or contradictory: What do you think is the matter with you, or what worries you the most?

PEDIATRIC VARIATIONS

Building the History

These are only guidelines; you are free to modify and add as the needs of your patients and your judgment dictate.

Chief Concern

A guardian or other responsible adult will generally be the major resource. When age permits, the child should be involved as much as possible. Remember that every chief concern has the potential of an underlying concern. What really led to your visit? Was it just the sore throat?

Reliability

Note relationship to patient of person who is the resource for history, and record your impression of the reliability of that person as a historian.

History of Present Illness

Be sure to give a clear chronologic sequence to the story.

Medical History

In general, the age of the patient and the nature of the problem will guide your approach. Clearly, in a continuing relationship, much of what is to be known will already have been recorded. Certainly, different aspects of the history require varying emphasis depending on the nature of the immediate problem. Certain specifics will command attention, including the following:

- Pregnant person's health:
  - Infectious disease; give approximate gestational month
  - Weight gain/edema
  - Hypertension

- Proteinuria
- Bleeding; approximate time
- Eclampsia, threat of eclampsia
- Special or unusual diet or dietary practices
- Medications (hormones, vitamins)
- Quality of fetal movements, time of onset
- Radiation exposure
- Prenatal care/consistency
- Birth and perinatal experience:
  - Duration of pregnancy
  - Delivery site
  - Labor: spontaneous/induced, duration, anesthesia, complications
  - Delivery: presentation; forceps/spontaneous; complications
  - Condition at birth: time of onset of cry; Apgar scores, if available
  - Birth weight and, if available, length and head circumference
- Neonatal period:
  - Hospital experience: length of stay, feeding experience, oxygen needs, vigor, color (jaundice, cyanosis), cry. Did infant go home with mother?
  - First month of life: color (jaundice), feeding, vigor, any suggestion of illness or untoward event
- Feeding:
  - Bottle or breast: any changes and why; type of formula, amounts offered/taken, feeding frequency; weight gain
  - Present diet and appetite: introduction of solids, current routine and frequency, age weaned from bottle or breast, daily intake of milk, food preferences, ability to feed self; elaborate on any feeding problems

Development

Guidelines suggested in Chapter 5 are complementary to the milestones detailed in the following lists. Those included in this section are commonly used. Photographs also may occasionally be of some help. **NOTE:** It is important to define the growth and developmental status of each child regardless of the particular concern. That status will inform your understanding of the child, and of the particular problem, and will facilitate the institution of a management plan.
- Age when:
  - Held head erect while held in sitting position
  - Sat alone, unsupported

- Walked alone
  - Talked in sentences
  - Toilet trained
- School: grade, performance, learning and social problems
- Dentition: ages for first teeth, loss of deciduous teeth, first permanent teeth
- Growth: height and weight at different ages, changes in rate of growth or weight gain or loss
- Sexual: present status (e.g., in female patients, time of breast development, nipples, pubic hair, description of menses; in male patients, development of pubic hair, voice change, acne, emissions). Follow Tanner stages of physical sexual maturity development guides.

Family History

- Maternal gestational history: all pregnancies with status of each, including date, age, cause of death of all deceased siblings, and dates and duration of pregnancy in the case of miscarriages; mother's health during pregnancy
- Age of parents at birth of patient
- Are parents related to each other in any way?

Personal and Social History

- Personal status:
  - School adjustment
  - Nail biting
  - Thumb sucking
  - Breath-holding
  - Temper tantrums
  - Pica
  - Tics
  - Rituals
- Home conditions:
  - Parental occupation(s)
  - Principal caretaker(s) of patient
  - Food preparation, routine, family preferences (e.g., vegetarianism), who does preparing
  - Adequacy of clothing
  - Dependency on relief or social agencies
  - Number of persons and rooms in house or apartment
  - Sleeping routines and sleep arrangements for child

Review of Systems (Some Suggested Additional Questions or Particular Concerns)

- Ears: otitis media (frequency, laterality)
- Nose: snoring, mouth breathing
- Teeth: dental care
- Genitourinary: nature of urinary stream, forceful or a dribble
- Skin, hair, nails: eczema or seborrhea

OLDER ADULT VARIATIONS

Functional Assessment

- Activities of daily living (ADLs): ability to independently perform or amount of assistance needed with the following:
  - Bathing
  - Dressing
  - Toileting
  - Transfers
  - Grooming
  - Feeding
- Instrumental ADLs: ability to independently perform or amount of assistance needed with the following:
  - Administering own medication
  - Grocery shopping
  - Preparing meals
  - Using the telephone
  - Driving and transportation
  - Handling own finances
  - Housekeeping
  - Laundry
- Risk for falls: falls in the past 6 months or year; use of rugs at home
- Cognitive functioning: see Chapter 4

2 Vital Signs and Pain Assessment

Equipment

- Thermometer
- Sphygmomanometer
- Stethoscope
- Pain scales

EXAMINATION

TECHNIQUES	FINDINGS

Vital Signs

Temperature

Take the temperature with an oral, tympanic, axillary, temporal, or rectal thermometer.

EXPECTED: Temperature range of 97.2°F to 99.9°F (36.2°C to 37.7°C).
UNEXPECTED: Fever, hypothermia.

Pulse rate

Palpate the radial or brachial pulse to count the heart rate for 30 seconds and multiply by 2. Note the contour and amplitude of the pulsation. See Chapter 12 for rhythm assessment.

EXPECTED: Rate 60 to 90 beats/min, average 70, regular rhythm.
UNEXPECTED: Bradycardia, tachycardia, irregular rhythm.

Palpating the radial pulse.

TECHNIQUES   FINDINGS

Respiratory rate

Assess the respiratory rate for 30 seconds and multiply by 2. See Chapter 10 to assess the pattern of respirations.

EXPECTED: Breathing easy, regular, without distress. Pattern even. Rate 12 to 20 respirations/min. Ratio of respirations to heartbeats about 1:4.
UNEXPECTED: Tachypnea, bradypnea, dyspnea.

Blood pressure

Measure in both arms at least once annually. Patient's arm should be slightly flexed and positioned or held at the level of the heart.

EXPECTED: Less than 120 mm Hg systolic and less than 80 mm Hg diastolic, with pulse pressure of 30 to 40 mm Hg (sometimes to 50 mm Hg). Reading between arms may vary by as much as 10 mm Hg. Prehypertension is now defined as a blood pressure between 120 and 139 mm Hg systolic or 80 and 89 mm Hg diastolic.
UNEXPECTED: Hypertension (see the following table). Unusually low readings should be evaluated for clinical significance.

Classification of Blood Pressure for Adults Aged 18 Years and Older*

CATEGORY	SYSTOLIC (MM HG)		DIASTOLIC (MM HG)
Optimal	<120	and	<80
Prehypertension	120-139	or	80-89
Hypertension†			
Stage 1	140-159	or	90-99
Stage 2	≥160	or	≥100

From National Institutes of Health Publication No. 04-5320, 2004.

*Not taking antihypertensive drugs and not acutely ill. When systolic and diastolic blood pressures fall into different categories, the higher category should be selected to classify the individual's blood pressure status. For example, 160/92 mm Hg should be classified as stage 2 hypertension. In addition to classifying stages of hypertension on the basis of average blood pressure levels, clinicians should specify presence or absence of target organ disease and additional risk factors.

†Based on the average of two or more readings taken at each of two or more visits after an initial screening.

TECHNIQUES

FINDINGS

Pain Assessment

Explain how to use the pain assessment tool. See the following figures. Ask the patient to indicate the pain level at each site and then to describe the pain characteristics. Observe for pain behaviors.

EXPECTED: The patient does not have pain or the painful condition is well managed.
UNEXPECTED: Pain level greater than 3. Pain characteristics such as stabbing, sharp, dull, or aching. Documented pain rating. Behaviors indicating pain such as guarding, facial grimace or other expression of pain, groaning, or rubbing or holding painful site.

Pain Assessment Tools

Numeric Pain Intensity Scale.

Visual analog scale.

Wong-Baker FACES pain rating scale. (From Hockenberry MJ, Wilson D, Rodgers CC: Wong's essentials of pediatric nursing, ed 10, St. Louis, 2017, Elsevier.)

EXAMINATION

TECHNIQUES
FINDINGS

VITAL SIGNS AND PAIN ASSESSMENT

Pulse Rate

Palpate the pulse or use a stethoscope to auscultate the apical pulse.

EXPECTED:

Age	Beats/min
Newborn	120-170
1 year	80-160
3 years	80-120
6 years	75-115
10 years	70-110

Respiratory Rate

Observe abdominal rise to count the respiratory rate in infants and toddlers.

EXPECTED:

Age	Respirations/min
Newborn	24-50
1 year	20-40
3 years	20-30
6 years	16-22
10 years	16-20
17 years	12-20

UNEXPECTED: Sustained rate higher or lower than expected range.

Measure the Blood Pressure

Select the appropriate size cuff to measure the infant's or child's blood pressure.
- The cuff width should cover approximately 70% of the distance between the shoulder and the elbow.
- The bladder length should be 80% to 100% of the upper arm circumference, and the bladder width should be at least 40% of the arm circumference at the midpoint of the acromion-olecranon distance.

EXPECTED: For children aged ≥1 year, <90th percentile for age, gender, and height percentile (see tables on pp. 14-17). UNEXPECTED: ≥90th percentile for age, gender, and height percentile is an elevated blood pressure. ≥95th percentile is Stage 1 hypertension.

Blood Pressure Levels for the 90th and 95th Percentiles of Blood Pressure for Boys 1 to 17 Years of Age by Percentile of Height

AGE, YEARS	BLOOD PRESSURE PERCENTILE*	SYSTOLIC BLOOD PRESSURE BY PERCENTILE OF HEIGHT, MM HG†							DIASTOLIC BLOOD PRESSURE BY PERCENTILE OF HEIGHT, MM HG†						
		5TH	10TH	25TH	50TH	75TH	90TH	95TH	5TH	10TH	25TH	50TH	75TH	90TH	95TH
1	90th	98	99	99	100	100	101	101	52	52	53	53	54	54	54
	95th	102	102	103	103	104	105	105	54	54	55	55	56	57	57
2	90th	100	100	101	102	103	103	104	55	55	56	56	57	58	58
	95th	104	105	105	106	107	107	108	57	58	58	59	60	61	61
3	90th	101	102	102	103	104	105	105	58	58	59	59	60	61	61
	95th	106	106	107	107	108	109	109	60	61	61	62	63	64	64
4	90th	102	103	104	105	105	106	107	60	61	62	62	63	64	64
	95th	107	107	108	108	109	110	110	63	64	65	66	67	67	68
5	90th	103	104	105	106	107	108	108	63	64	65	65	66	67	67
	95th	107	108	109	109	110	111	112	66	67	68	69	70	71	71
6	90th	105	105	106	107	109	110	110	66	66	67	68	68	69	69
	95th	108	109	110	111	112	113	114	69	70	70	71	72	72	73
7	90th	106	107	108	109	110	111	111	68	68	69	70	70	71	71
	95th	110	110	111	112	114	115	116	71	71	72	73	73	74	74
8	90th	107	107	108	110	111	112	112	69	70	70	71	72	72	73
	95th	111	112	112	114	115	116	117	72	73	73	74	75	75	75

Age (y)	BP Percentile*	SBP (mm Hg) Height Percentile†							DBP (mm Hg) Height Percentile†						
9	90th	107	108	109	110	112	113	114	70	71	72	73	74	74	74
	95th	112	112	113	115	116	118	119	74	74	75	76	76	77	77
10	90th	108	109	111	112	113	115	116	72	73	74	74	75	76	76
	95th	112	113	114	116	118	118	121	76	76	77	77	78	78	78
11	90th	110	111	112	114	116	117	118	74	74	75	75	75	76	76
	95th	114	114	116	118	120	123	124	77	77	78	78	78	79	81
12	90th	113	114	115	117	119	121	122	75	75	75	75	76	76	76
	95th	116	117	118	121	124	126	128	78	78	78	78	79	79	79
13	90th	115	116	118	121	124	124	126	74	74	75	75	76	76	76
	95th	119	120	122	125	128	130	131	78	78	78	78	80	80	81
14	90th	119	120	123	126	127	128	129	74	74	75	77	78	78	80
	95th	123	125	127	130	132	133	134	77	78	79	81	82	83	84
15	90th	123	124	126	128	129	130	130	75	76	78	79	80	80	81
	95th	127	129	131	132	134	135	135	78	79	81	83	84	84	85
16	90th	126	127	128	129	131	131	132	77	78	79	80	81	82	82
	95th	130	131	133	134	135	136	137	80	81	83	84	85	86	86
17	90th	128	129	130	131	132	133	134	78	79	80	81	82	82	83
	95th	132	133	134	135	137	138	138	81	82	83	85	86	86	87

Adapted from: Flynn, J. T., Kaelber, D. C., Baker-Smith, C. M., et al. (2017). Clinical practice guideline for screening and management of high blood pressure in children and adolescents. *Pediatrics, 140*(3):e20171904.

*Blood pressure percentile was determined by a single measurement.

†Height percentile was determined by standard growth curves.

VITAL SIGNS AND PAIN ASSESSMENT

Blood Pressure Levels for the 90th and 95th Percentiles of Blood Pressure for Girls 1 to 17 Years of Age by Percentile of Height

AGE, YEARS	BLOOD PRESSURE PERCENTILE*	SYSTOLIC BLOOD PRESSURE BY PERCENTILE OF HEIGHT, MM HG†							DIASTOLIC BLOOD PRESSURE BY PERCENTILE OF HEIGHT, MM HG†						
		5TH	10TH	25TH	50TH	75TH	90TH	95TH	5TH	10TH	25TH	50TH	75TH	90TH	95TH
1	90th	98	99	99	100	101	102	102	54	55	56	56	57	58	58
	95th	101	102	102	103	104	105	105	59	59	60	60	61	62	62
2	90th	101	101	102	103	104	105	106	58	58	59	60	61	62	62
	95th	104	105	106	106	107	108	109	62	63	63	64	65	66	66
3	90th	102	103	104	104	105	106	107	60	61	61	62	63	64	65
	95th	106	106	107	108	109	110	110	64	65	65	66	67	68	69
4	90th	103	104	105	106	107	108	108	62	63	64	65	66	67	67
	95th	107	108	109	109	110	111	112	66	67	68	69	70	71	71
5	90th	104	105	106	107	108	109	110	64	65	66	67	68	69	70
	95th	108	109	109	110	111	112	113	68	69	70	71	72	73	73
6	90th	105	106	107	108	109	110	111	67	67	68	69	70	71	71
	95th	109	109	110	111	112	113	114	70	71	72	72	73	74	74
7	90th	106	106	107	109	110	111	112	68	68	69	70	71	72	72
	95th	109	110	111	112	113	114	115	72	72	73	73	74	74	75
8	90th	107	107	108	110	111	112	113	69	70	71	72	72	73	73
	95th	110	111	112	113	115	116	117	72	73	74	74	75	75	75

Age	BP Percentile														
9	90th	108	108	109	111	112	113	114	71	71	72	73	73	73	73
	95th	112	112	113	114	116	117	118	74	74	75	75	75	75	75
10	90th	109	110	111	112	113	115	116	72	73	73	73	73	73	73
	95th	113	114	114	116	117	119	120	75	75	76	76	76	76	76
11	90th	111	112	113	114	116	118	120	74	74	74	74	74	75	75
	95th	115	116	117	118	120	123	124	76	77	77	77	77	77	77
12	90th	114	115	116	118	120	122	122	75	75	75	75	76	76	76
	95th	118	119	120	122	124	125	126	78	78	78	78	79	79	79
13	90th	116	117	119	121	122	123	123	75	75	75	76	76	76	76
	95th	121	122	123	124	126	126	127	79	79	79	79	80	81	81
14	90th	118	118	120	122	123	123	123	76	76	76	76	77	77	77
	95th	123	123	124	125	126	127	127	80	80	80	80	81	82	82
15	90th	118	119	121	122	123	123	124	76	76	76	77	77	77	78
	95th	124	124	125	126	127	128	128	80	80	80	81	82	82	82
16	90th	119	120	122	122	123	124	124	76	76	76	77	78	78	78
	95th	124	125	125	127	127	128	128	80	80	80	81	82	82	82
17	90th	120	121	123	124	124	125	125	76	76	77	77	78	78	78
	95th	125	125	126	127	128	128	128	80	80	80	81	82	82	82

Adapted From: Flynn, J. T., Kaelber, D. C., Baker-Smith, C. M., et al. (2017). Clinical practice guideline for screening and management of high blood pressure in children and adolescents. Pediatrics, 140(3):e20171904.

*Blood pressure percentile was determined by a single measurement.

†Height percentile was determined by standard growth curves.

VITAL SIGNS AND PAIN ASSESSMENT

TECHNIQUES   FINDINGS

Pain Assessment

Observe for pain behaviors using a tool such as the Face, Legs, Activity, Cry, and Consolability (FLACC) Behavioral Pain Assessment Scale when the child is unable to use a self-report pain assessment tool. See the following FLACC figure.

UNEXPECTED: The child has pain behaviors such as crying, posturing, restlessness, or facial grimace and is difficult to comfort.

	SCORING		
CATEGORIES	0	1	2
Face	No particular expression or smile	Occasional grimace or frown; withdrawn, disinterested	Frequent to constant frown, clenched jaw, quivering chin
Legs	Normal position or relaxed	Uneasy, restless, tense	Kicking or legs drawn up
Activity	Lying quietly, normal position, moves easily	Squirming, shifting back and forth, tense	Arched, rigid, or jerking
Cry	No cry (awake or asleep)	Moans or whimpers, occasional complaint	Crying steadily, screams or sobs; frequent complaints
Consolability	Content, relaxed	Reassured by occasional touching, hugging, or being talked to; distractable	Difficult to console or comfort

Guidelines for Scoring the FLACC

Face
Score 0 if the patient has a relaxed face, makes eye contact, shows interest in surroundings.
Score 1 if the patient has a worried facial expression, with eyebrows lowered, eyes partially closed, cheeks raised, mouth pursed.
Score 2 if the patient has deep furrows in the forehead, closed eyes, an open mouth, deep lines around nose and lips.

Legs
Score 0 if the muscle tone and motion in the limbs are normal.
Score 1 if patient has increased tone, rigidity, or tension; if there is intermittent flexion or extension of the limbs.
Score 2 if patient has hypertonicity, the legs are pulled tight, there is exaggerated flexion or extension of the limbs, tremors.

Activity
Score 0 if the patient moves easily and freely, normal activity or restrictions.
Score 1 if the patient shifts positions, appears hesitant to move, demonstrates guarding, a tense torso, pressure on a body part.
Score 2 if the patient is in a fixed position, rocking; demonstrates side-to-side head movement or rubbing of a body part.

Cry
Score 0 if the patient has no cry or moan, awake or asleep.
Score 1 if the patient has occasional moans, cries, whimpers, sighs.
Score 2 if the patient has frequent or continuous moans, cries, grunts.

Consolability
Score 0 if the patient is calm and does not require consoling.
Score 1 if the patient responds to comfort by touching or talking in 30 seconds to 1 minute.
Score 2 if the patient requires constant comforting or is inconsolable.

Interpreting the Behavioral Score
Each category is scored on the 0–2 scale, which results in a total score of 0–10.

0 = Relaxed and comfortable   4–6 = Moderate pain
1–3 = Mild discomfort   7–10 = Severe discomfort or pain or both

Face, Legs, Activity, Cry, and Consolability (FLACC) Behavioral Pain Assessment Scale for nonverbal children. (From Merkel SI, et al: The FLACC: A behavioral scale for scoring postoperative pain in young children, Pediatr Nurs 23(2):293–297, 1997.)

TECHNIQUES   FINDINGS

For nonverbal older adults, use the Pain Assessment in Advanced Dementia Scale to assess pain behaviors.

	0	1	2	Score
Breathing Independent of vocalization	Normal	Occasional labored breathing. Short period of hyperventilation.	Noisy labored breathing. Long period of hyperventilation. Cheyne-Stokes respirations.	
Negative vocalization	None	Occasional moan or groan. Low-level speech with a negative or disapproving quality.	Repeated troubled calling out. Loud moaning or groaning. Crying.	
Facial expression	Smiling, or inexpressive	Sad. Frightened. Frown.	Facial grimacing.	
Body language	Relaxed	Tense. Distressed pacing. Fidgeting.	Rigid. Fists clenched. Knees pulled up. Pulling or pushing away. Striking out.	
Consolability	No need to console	Distracted or reassured by voice or touch.	Unable to console, distract, or reassure.	
			TOTAL	

Pain Assessment in Advanced Dementia (PAINAD) Scale. Note: Total scores range from 0 to 10, when scoring 0, 1, or 2 for each item. A score of 0 = no observable pain and 10 = highest observable pain. (From Warden V, Hurley AC, and Volicer L: Development and psychometric evaluation of the Pain Assessment in Advanced Dementia (PAINAD) Scale, Journal of the American Medical Directors Association, 4:9–15, 2003.)

VITAL SIGNS AND PAIN ASSESSMENT

3   Mental Status

Equipment

- Familiar objects (coins, keys, paper clips)
- Paper and pencil

EXAMINATION

Perform the mental status examination throughout the patient interaction. Focus on the patient's alertness, orientation, mood, and cognition or complex mental processes (learning, perceiving, decision making, and memory). Use a mental status screening examination for health visits when no cognitive, emotional, or behavioral problems are apparent. Information is generally observed during the history in the following areas:

APPEARANCE AND BEHAVIOR	EMOTIONAL STABILITY
Grooming	Mood and feelings
Emotional status	Thought process and content
Body language	

COGNITIVE ABILITIES	SPEECH AND LANGUAGE
State of consciousness	Voice quality
Memory	Articulation
Attention span	Comprehension
Judgment	Coherence
	Ability to communicate

Note any reliance on another adult to answer questions. When concerned about any of the patient's responses or behaviors, ask a family member if the patient has had any problems with memory or cognitive function, such as forgetting important appointments or events, paying bills, and taking medications. Additionally determine if the patient shops independently for food or clothing, gets lost while walking or driving, and makes decisions about daily life.

TECHNIQUE	FINDINGS

Mental Status and Speech Patterns
Observe physical appearance and behavior

- *Grooming*

UNEXPECTED: Poor hygiene; lack of concern with appearance; or inappropriate dress for season, gender, or occasion in previously well-groomed patient.

- *Emotional status*

EXPECTED: Usually friendly and cooperative; expresses concern appropriate for emotional content of topics discussed.
UNEXPECTED: Behavior conveys carelessness, apathy, loss of sympathetic responses, unusual docility, rage reactions, agitation, or excessive irritability.

- *Body language*

EXPECTED: Erect posture and eye contact (if culturally appropriate).
UNEXPECTED: Slumped posture, lack of facial expression, excessively energetic movements, or constantly watchful eyes.

- *State of consciousness*

EXPECTED: Oriented to person, place, and time; appropriate responses to questions and environmental stimuli.
UNEXPECTED: Disoriented to time, place, or person. Verbal response is confused, incoherent, or inappropriate, or there is no verbal response.

Investigate Cognitive Abilities

- *Mini-Cog*
Ask patient to remember and immediately repeat three unrelated words (e.g., *red, plate,* and *milk*). Ask patient to draw a clock face with numbers, then draw the clock hands pointing to the time you specify. Allow 3 minutes. Ask the patient to repeat the three words. Score 1 point for each word recalled.

EXPECTED: All three words are remembered, and the clock face has all numbers in proper position and hands pointing to the specified time.
UNEXPECTED: A score of ≤2 may indicate dementia.

MENTAL STATUS

TECHNIQUE	FINDINGS

Score 2 points when all numbers of the clock face are near the rim, in correct sequence, and hands point to the specified time. Total of 5 points (Milian et al, 2012).

From Stern T, Fricchione G, et al.: Massachusetts General Hospital Handbook of General Hospital Psychiatry. ed 6, 2010, Elsevier, Philadelphia.)

• *Montreal Cognitive Assessment*
This is a more extensive test of memory recall and executive functioning, taking 10 to 20 minutes to administer. It helps identify mild cognitive impairment (Dong et al, 2012). See www.mocatest.org to access the screening tool.

EXPECTED: Score of ≥20.
UNEXPECTED: Score ≤20 points indicates multiple domain mild cognitive impairment that is associated with a higher risk for of dementia.

• *Analogies*
Ask patient to describe analogies: first simple, then more complex
  • What is similar about peaches and lemons, oceans and lakes, trumpet and flute?
  • An engine is to an airplane as an oar is to a _____?
  • What is different about a magazine and a cookbook, or a bush and a tree?

EXPECTED: Correct responses when patient has average intelligence.
UNEXPECTED: Unable to describe similarities or differences.

• *Abstract reasoning*
Ask patient to explain meaning of fable, proverb, or metaphor.
  • A stitch in time saves nine.
  • A bird in the hand is worth two in the bush.
  • A rolling stone gathers no moss.

EXPECTED: Adequate interpretation when patient has average intelligence.
UNEXPECTED: Unable to give adequate explanation.

TECHNIQUE	FINDINGS

• *Arithmetic calculations*
Ask patient to perform simple calculations without paper and pencil.
   • 50 – 7, – 7, – 7, etc., until answer is 8.
   • 50 + 8, + 8, + 8, etc., until answer is 98.
	EXPECTED: Able to complete with few errors within a minute.
	UNEXPECTED: Unable to perform calculations.

• *Writing ability* Ask patient to write name and address or a phrase you dictate (or if literacy is a problem, draw figures—triangle, circle, square, flower, house, clockface).	UNEXPECTED: Omission or addition of letters, syllables, or words; mirror writing; or uncoordinated writing (or figure drawings).
• *Execution of motor skills* Ask patient to do a motor task such as combing hair or putting on lipstick.	UNEXPECTED: Inability to complete a task that is not related to paralysis.
• *Memory* *Immediate recall or new learning:* Ask patient to listen to, then repeat, a sentence or series of numbers. *Recent memory:* Ask the patient to remember the four or five objects shown, or give a visually impaired patient four unrelated words with distinct sounds to remember (carpet, iris, bench, fortune). In 10 minutes, ask patient to list objects. *Remote memory:* Ask patient about verifiable past events (e.g., mother's maiden name, name of high school, subject of common knowledge).	EXPECTED: *Immediate recall:* Able to repeat sentence or numbers (five to eight numbers forward, four to six numbers backward). *Recent memory:* Able to remember test objects. *Remote memory:* Able to recall verifiable past events. UNEXPECTED: Impaired memory. Loss of immediate and recent memory with retention of remote memory.

TECHNIQUE	FINDINGS
• *Attention span* Ask patient to follow a series of short commands (e.g., take off all clothes, put on patient gown, sit on examining table), or spell *world* forward and backward. Arithmetic calculation is another test of attention span.	EXPECTED: Responds to directions appropriately. UNEXPECTED: Easy distraction or confusion, negativism.

• *Judgment*
Explore:
  • How patient meets social and family obligations, patient's future plans.
  • Patient's solutions to hypothetical situations (e.g., found stamped envelope or was stopped by police for running a red light).
	EXPECTED: Able to evaluate situation and provide appropriate response; managing family and business affairs appropriately.
	UNEXPECTED: Response indicating hazardous behavior or inappropriate action.

Observe speech and language

• *Voice quality*	EXPECTED: Uses inflections, speaks clearly and strongly, is able to increase voice volume and pitch. UNEXPECTED: Difficulty or discomfort making laryngeal speech sounds or varying volume, quality, or pitch of speech.
• *Articulation*	EXPECTED: Proper pronunciation of consonants; fluent and rhythmic speech; easily expresses thoughts. UNEXPECTED: Imperfect or slurring pronunciation, difficulty articulating single speech sound, or speech with hesitancy, stuttering, or repetitions.

TECHNIQUE	FINDINGS
• *Comprehension*	EXPECTED: Able to follow simple one- and two-step instructions.
• *Coherence*	EXPECTED: Able to clearly convey intentions or perceptions. UNEXPECTED: Circumlocutions, perseveration, flight of ideas or loosening of associations between thoughts, gibberish, neologisms, clang association, echolalia, or unusual sounds may be associated with a psychiatric disorder. Hesitations, omissions, inappropriate word substitutions, circumlocutions, neologisms, disturbance of rhythm or words in sequence may be signs of aphasia.

MENTAL STATUS

Evaluate emotional stability

• *Mood and feelings* Ask patient how he or she feels, whether feelings are a problem in daily life, and whether he or she has particularly difficult times or experiences.	EXPECTED: Expresses appropriate feelings for the situation. UNEXPECTED: Unresponsiveness, hopelessness, agitation, aggression, anger, euphoria, irritability, or wide mood swings.
• *Depression screening questions* • Over the past 2 weeks, have you felt down, depressed, or hopeless? • Over the past 2 weeks, have you felt little interest or pleasure in doing things?	EXPECTED: Negative response to one or both questions. UNEXPECTED: Positive response to both questions indicates a need to ask more questions about depression symptoms of fatigue, restlessness, and poor concentration. The Patient Health Questionnaire 9 (PHQ-9) may be used for further assessment. See www.phqscreeners.com for access to the tool.

MENTAL STATUS

TECHNIQUE   FINDINGS

Ask the patient to choose the best answer for how he or she felt over the previous week.

1. Are you basically satisfied with your life?	YES / NO
2. Have you dropped many of your activities and interests?	YES / NO
3. Do you feel that your life is empty?	YES / NO
4. Do you often get bored?	YES / NO
5. Are you in good spirits most of the time?	YES / NO
6. Are you afraid that something bad is going to happen to you?	YES / NO
7. Do you feel happy most of the time?	YES / NO
8. Do you feel helpless?	YES / NO
9. Do you prefer to stay at home, rather than going out and doing new things?	YES / NO
10. Do you feel you have more problems with memory than most?	YES / NO
11. Do you think it is wonderful to be alive now?	YES / NO
12. Do you feel pretty worthless the way you are now?	YES / NO
13. Do you feel full of energy?	YES / NO
14. Do you feel that your situation is hopeless?	YES / NO
15. Do you think most people are better off than you are?	YES / NO

Correct responses are the following:
 Yes for questions 2, 3, 4, 6, 8, 9, 10, 12, 14, and 15.
 No for questions 1, 5, 7, 11, and 13.
Give one point for each correct answer. A score greater than five suggests depression.
Geriatric Depression Scale. (From Sheikh JI, Yesavage JA: Geriatric depression scale: recent evidence and development of a shorter version, Clin Gerontol 5:165-172, 1986.)

- *Thought process and content*
  - Ask patient about obsessive thoughts relating to making decisions, fears, or guilt.
  - Ask patient about the need to compulsively repeat actions, check, and recheck (or observe the patient's actions).
  - Observe sequence, logic, coherence, and relevance of topics.
  - Does patient have delusions (of grandeur, of being controlled by external force)? Does the patient feel watched, followed, persecuted, or paranoid?

EXPECTED: Patient's thought processes can be followed, and ideas expressed are logical and goal directed.
UNEXPECTED: Illogical or unrealistic thought processes; blocking or disturbance in stream of thinking. Obsessive thought content, compulsive behavior, phobias, anxieties that interfere with daily life or are disabling; delusions.

TECHNIQUE	FINDINGS
• *Perceptual distortions and hallucinations* 　• Ask patient about any sensations you believe are not caused by external stimuli. 　• Find out when these experiences occur.	UNEXPECTED: Sensory hallucinations—hears voices, sees vivid images or shadowy figures, smells offensive odors, feels worms crawling on skin.

MENTAL STATUS

AIDS TO DIFFERENTIAL DIAGNOSIS

SUBJECTIVE DATA	OBJECTIVE DATA
Dementia	
Forgets significant events; gets lost in familiar areas; unable to manage shopping, food preparation, medications; mood changes (depression, uncharacteristic anger, anxiety, or agitation); apathy; behavior changes (e.g., impulsiveness, socially inappropriate dress).	Impaired memory, social and occupational functioning, and activities of daily living; impaired use of language; impaired executive functioning; progressive deterioration in cognitive function.
Delirium	
Sudden impairment of memory and attentiveness, mood swings, increased or decreased activity.	Altered consciousness; fearful, suspicious; rambling and irrelevant conversation, illogical flow of ideas. Misperceptions, illusions, hallucinations, and delusions; symptoms increase and decrease during the day.
Depression	
Feels sad, hopeless, worthless; guilt, loss of pleasure or interest; loss of energy, insomnia or excessive sleeping; increased or decreased appetite. May have had a loss, change in health status, stressful life event.	Altered mood and affect with extreme sadness, anxiety, irritability; impaired concentration, reduced attention span, indecisiveness, slower thought processes.

MENTAL STATUS

SUBJECTIVE DATA	OBJECTIVE DATA
Mania	
Persistently elevated and expansive mood, hyperactivity, overconfidence, exaggerated view of own abilities, hyperactivity, racing thoughts.	Increased talkativeness or pressure to keep talking with excessive rhyming, puns, or flight of ideas; impaired attention, judgment, social, occupational, and interpersonal functioning; grandiose or persecutory delusions; hypersexual behavior.
Anxiety Disorder	
Anxiety or fear that interferes with personal, social, occupational functioning. Panic attacks (palpitations, sweating, shaking, dizziness, nausea, chest pain, abdominal distress); nightmares; flashbacks; poor concentration; sleeps poorly.	Tachycardia, diaphoresis, tremors, impaired attention, ritualized acts performed compulsively.

Sample Documentation

Subjective. A 66-year-old woman accompanied by spouse who expresses concern about his wife's memory loss. She got lost in the local shopping mall last week. Previously was a good cook, but over the last few months either does not have necessary ingredients or has difficulty following recipes. Needs help to take correct daily medications. Dresses and undresses self but needs help to select clothes to wear. Patient recognizes all family members and social contacts and is able to talk with them.

Objective. Pleasant woman with clear speech, responds to simple questions correctly. Turns to spouse frequently for answers to some history questions. Follows one-step directions but needs reminder with two-step directions. Immediate and recent memory impaired, but remote memory is intact. Arithmetic calculation impaired. Mini-Cog score = 2.

PEDIATRIC VARIATIONS

EXAMINATION

TECHNIQUE	FINDINGS
Mental Status	
Use parent's impression of infant's responsiveness to guide your assessment. Questionnaires completed by parents (e.g., Ages and Stages Questionnaire or Parent's Evaluation of Developmental Status) are effective screening tools.	EXPECTED: Infant responds appropriately to parent's voice, is attentive, comforts easily. Social smile can be elicited; babbling or cooing or language appropriate for age. Child follows simple directions. UNEXPECTED: Nonresponsive, inconsolable, combative, lethargic.

AIDS TO DIFFERENTIAL DIAGNOSIS

SUBJECTIVE DATA	OBJECTIVE DATA
Intellectual Disability	
Delayed motor, speech, and language development.	Delayed developmental milestones, impaired cognitive functioning and short-term memory; poor academic performance; lack of motivation.
Autism	
Does not make eye contact or point to share experiences with others; resists being held or touched; odd and repetitive behaviors, ritualized play, preoccupation with objects; motor development appropriate for age.	Impaired social interactions and language, odd intonation to speech, pronoun reversal, nonsensical rhyming; lacks awareness of others.
Attention-Deficit/Hyperactivity	
Short attention span, easily distracted, fidgets and squirms, often moving, disruptive behavior, talks excessively, temper outbursts; has problems in more than one setting.	Increased motor activity, difficulty organizing tasks, poor school performance.

4   Growth and Nutrition

Equipment

- Standing platform scale with height attachment
- Measuring tape with millimeter markings
- Infant scale
- Recumbent measuring device (for infants)
- Stature measuring device (for children)
- Calculator

EXAMINATION

TECHNIQUE	FINDINGS

Anthropometrics

Measure height and weight

- For weight, ask the patient to remove excess clothing and shoes. Have the patient stand in the middle of the scale platform and note the digital reading.

  EXPECTED: *Women:* 100 pounds for first 5 feet, plus 5 pounds for each inch thereafter. *Men:* 106 pounds for first 5 feet, plus 6 pounds for each inch thereafter.

- For height, have the patient stand erect with his or her back to the stature-measuring device. Pull up the height attachment and position the headpiece on the top of the head. Make the reading at the nearest centimeter or half inch.

- Calculate percent weight change:

$$\left(\frac{\text{Usual weight} - \text{Current weight}}{\text{Usual weight}}\right) \times 100$$

  UNEXPECTED: Weight loss that equals or exceeds 1% to 2% in 1 week, 5% in 1 month, 7.5% in 3 months, 10% in 6 months.

TECHNIQUE	FINDINGS

- Calculate body mass index (BMI) kg/m^2 or calculate using pounds by:

$$\frac{(\text{Weight in pounds} \times 703)}{(\text{Height in inches} \times \text{Height in inches})}$$

EXPECTED: 18.5–24.9 for men and women.
UNEXPECTED: BMI <18.5 is classified as undernutrition. BMI 25–29.9 is classified as overweight. BMI ≥30 is obesity.

Measure waist circumference

Indicator of visceral fat. Using a tape measure with millimeter markings, measure waist at high point of iliac crest when patient is standing and at minimal respiration.

EXPECTED: Waist circumference <40 inches for men and <35 inches for women.
UNEXPECTED: Measurements >40 inches in men and >35 inches in women are associated with increased risk for type 2 diabetes, hypertension, and cardiovascular disease.

Calculate waist-to-hip circumference ratio

Another measure of fat distribution. Using tape measure with millimeter markings, measure waist at a midpoint between the costal margin and the iliac crest. Then measure hip at the widest part of the gluteal region. Divide waist circumference by hip circumference to obtain the ratio.

EXPECTED: Ratio <0.9 in men and <0.8 in women.
UNEXPECTED: Ratios >1.0 in men and >0.85 in women indicate increased central fat distribution and increased risk for obesity-related disease.

TECHNIQUE	FINDINGS

Determine Diet Adequacy
24-hour diet recall and food diary

Ask patient to complete 24-hour food and beverage recall or a 3- or 4-day food diary that includes 1 weekend day. Ask specific questions about method of food preparation, portion sizes, amount of sugar-sweetened beverages, and use of salt or other additives. The U.S. Department of Agriculture (USDA) ChooseMyPlate.gov website, based on the *2015-2020 Dietary Guidelines for Americans,* has useful web-based tools for tracking daily food and beverage intake by food groups (grains, vegetables, fruits, dairy and protein foods; www.supertracker.usda.gov/default.aspx).

EXPECTED: Plate of food should have half fruits and vegetables and half grains and protein. Recommended daily amounts of fruits, vegetables, grains, and protein is based on the individual's age, gender, weight, height. and level of physical activity. Recommendations can be found at http://www.choosemyplate.gov/MyPlate. ChooseMyPlate.gov emphasizes the following key messages:

- Focus on variety, amount, and nutrition.
- Choose foods and beverages with less saturated fat, sodium, and added sugars.
- Start with small changes to build healthier eating styles.
- Support healthy eating for everyone.

(From U.S. Department of Agriculture: ChooseMyPlate, 2017, http://www.choosemyplate.gov.)

TECHNIQUE	FINDINGS

Determine Nutritional Adequacy

Nutrition screening forms and web-based tools can be found on the USDA Food and Nutrition Information Center website (https://fnic.nal.usda.gov/).

AIDS TO DIFFERENTIAL DIAGNOSIS

SUBJECTIVE DATA	OBJECTIVE DATA

Obesity

Excessive caloric intake and high-fat foods, weight gain, decrease in physical exercise, recent life change or stress, medications, and disease processes.

Obesity-related symptoms or conditions include snoring and sleep apnea, shortness of breath, headaches, musculoskeletal symptoms, depression, irregular menses, polyuria, and polydipsia.

Body mass index (BMI)—overweight: 25-29.9, obesity: ≥30; excess fat located in breasts, buttocks, thighs; may have pale striae or acanthosis nigricans.

Anorexia Nervosa

Preoccupation with weight, excessive exercise and unusual eating habits including voluntary starvation, purging, vomiting, and weight control measures such as diet pills, use of laxatives, and diuretics.

Symptoms may include fatigue, dizziness, low energy, amenorrhea, weight loss or gain, constipation, bloating, abdominal discomfort, heartburn, intolerance to cold, palpitations, depression or irritability, decreased libido, and interrupted sleep.

Failure to maintain weight at 85% of ideal body weight for age and height, BMI ≤17.5; dry skin, lanugo hair, brittle nails, bradycardia, hypothermia, orthostatic hypotension, loss of muscle mass and subcutaneous fat; may have hypoglycemia, elevated liver enzymes, and thyroid hormone abnormalities.

SUBJECTIVE DATA	OBJECTIVE DATA
Bulimia	
Binge-eating episodes on average of 2 times per week followed by purging (e.g., vomiting, laxatives, diuretics); bloating, fullness, abdominal pain, heartburn.	Body weight may be normal, underweight, or overweight; knuckle calluses, dental enamel erosion, salivary gland enlargement; may have metabolic alkalosis, hypokalemia, or elevated salivary amylase.

Sample Documentation

Subjective. A 45-year-old man with steady weight gain over the past 5 years seeks nutrition counseling for weight-loss plan. Eats three full meals each day with snacking in between; eats breakfast and dinner at home, where wife prepares meals. Often eats lunch (fast foods) on the run. Sugar beverage intake: one or two cans of nondiet soda per day. No regular exercise. Has never kept a meal log. No change in lifestyle; moderate stress.

Objective. Height: 173 cm (68 inches); weight: 90.9 kg (200 pounds); BMI: 30.4; waist circumference: 42 inches; hip circumference: 41 inches; waist-to-hip ratio: 1.02.

PEDIATRIC VARIATIONS

EXAMINATION

TECHNIQUE	FINDINGS
Anthropometrics	
Growth assessment	
Measure the length of infants and children until age 24 months of age in a supine position on a measuring device. For children 2 years and older, obtain a standing height using a stature-measuring device (stadiometer). Weigh infants and children on a scale that measures grams and kilograms. Calculate body mass index (BMI) starting at 2 years of age. Use growth charts for pediatric patients (available at www.cdc.gov/growthcharts).	EXPECTED: Child is following a growth curve pattern for length or height and weight. Length or height and weight are approximately same percentiles. BMI is following a growth pattern expected for age. UNEXPECTED: • Underweight—BMI for age <5th percentile • At risk of overweight—BMI for age >85th percentile • Overweight—BMI for age >95th percentile

TECHNIQUE	FINDINGS

Measure head circumference

Wrap tape measure snugly around the head at the occipital protuberance and supraorbital prominence for infants and children younger than 2 years. Plot the measurement on the appropriate growth curve, and identify the child's percentile in comparison with the population standard. Compare measurements over time.

UNEXPECTED: Head circumference <3rd percentile or increasing in size at a rate faster than expected for age.

5 Skin, Hair, and Nails

Equipment

- Centimeter ruler (flexible, clear)
- Flashlight with transilluminator
- Handheld magnifying lens or dermatoscope (optional)
- Wood's lamp (to view fluorescing lesions)

EXAMINATION

TECHNIQUE	FINDINGS

Skin

Perform overall inspection of entire body

In particular, check areas not usually exposed and intertriginous surfaces.	EXPECTED: Skin color differences among body areas and between sun-exposed and non–sun-exposed areas. UNEXPECTED: Lesions.

Inspect skin of each body area and mucous membranes

• *Color/uniformity* Inspect sclerae, conjunctivae, buccal mucosa, tongue, lips, nail beds, and palms.	EXPECTED: General uniformity—dark brown to light tan, with pink or yellow overtones. Sun-darkened areas. Darker skin around knees and elbows. Calloused areas yellow. Knuckles darker and palms/soles lighter in dark-skinned patients. Vascular flush areas pink or red, especially with anxiety or excitement.

TECHNIQUE   FINDINGS

Spider angioma—
red central body
with radiating spi-
derlike legs that
blanch with pres-
sure to the central
body
Cause: Liver dis-
ease, vitamin B
deficiency, idio-
pathic

Purpura—red-
purple nonblanch-
able discoloration
greater than 0.5
cm diameter
Cause:
Intravascular
defects, infection

Venous star—
bluish spider, lin-
ear or irregularly
shaped; does not
blanch with pres-
sure
Cause: Increased
pressure in super-
ficial veins

Petechiae—red-
purple nonblanch-
able discoloration
less than 0.5 cm
diameter
Cause: Intravas-
cular defects, in-
fection

Telangiectasia—
fine, irregular red
line
Cause: Dilation of
capillaries

Ecchymoses—
red-purple non-
blanchable
discoloration of
variable size
Cause: Vascular
wall destruction,
trauma, vasculitis

Capillary heman-
gioma (nevus
flammeus)—red
irregular macular
patches
Cause: Dilation of
dermal capillaries

Cutaneous Color Changes

COLOR	CAUSE	DISTRIBUTION	SELECT CONDITIONS
Brown	Darkening of melanin pigment	Generalized	Pituitary, adrenal, liver disease Nevi, neurofibromatosis
White	Absence of pigmentation	Generalized Localized	Albinism Vitiligo
Red (erythema)	Increased cutaneous blood flow	Localized Generalized	Inflammation Fever, viral exanthems, urticaria
	Increased intravascular red blood cells	Generalized	Polycythemia

Continued

Cutaneous Color Changes—cont'd

COLOR	CAUSE	DISTRIBUTION	SELECT CONDITIONS
Yellow	Increased bile pigmentation (jaundice)	Generalized	Liver disease
	Increased carotene pigmentation	Generalized (except sclera)	Hypothyroidism, increased intake of vegetables containing carotene
	Decreased visibility of oxyhemoglobin	Generalized	Anemia, chronic renal disease
Blue	Increased unsaturated hemoglobin secondary to hypoxia	Lips, mouth, nail beds	Cardiovascular and pulmonary disease

TECHNIQUE	FINDINGS
	Pigmented nevi. Nonpigmented striae. Freckles. Birthmarks.
	UNEXPECTED: Dysplastic, precancerous, or cancerous nevi. Chloasma. Unpigmented skin. Generalized or localized color changes. Vascular skin lesions. Vascular changes.
• *Thickness*	EXPECTED: Thickness variations, with eyelids thinnest, areas of rubbing thickest. Calluses on hands and feet.
	UNEXPECTED: Atrophy. Hyperkeratosis. Corns.
• *Symmetry*	EXPECTED: Bilateral symmetry.
• *Hygiene*	EXPECTED: Clean.
Palpate skin	
• *Moisture*	EXPECTED: Minimal perspiration or oiliness. Increased perspiration (associated with activity, environment, obesity, anxiety, excitement) noticeable on palms, scalp, forehead, axillae.
	UNEXPECTED: Damp intertriginous areas.
• *Temperature* Palpate with dorsal surface of hand or fingers.	EXPECTED: Cool to warm. Bilateral symmetry.

TECHNIQUE	FINDINGS
• *Texture*	EXPECTED: Smooth, soft, and even. Roughness resulting from heavy clothing, cold weather, or soap. UNEXPECTED: Extensive or wide-spread roughness.
• *Turgor and mobility* Gently pinch skin on forearm or in sternal area, and release.	EXPECTED: Resilience. UNEXPECTED: Failure of skin to return to place quickly.

Inspect and palpate lesions

• *Size*
Measure all dimensions.

• *Shape*

• *Color*
Use Wood's lamp to distinguish fluorescing lesions.

• *Blanching*

• *Texture*
Transilluminate to determine presence of fluid.

• *Elevation/depression*

• *Pedunculation*

• *Exudate*
Note color, odor, amount, and consistency of lesion.

• *Configuration*
Check lesion for annular, grouped, linear, arciform, or diffuse arrangement.

• *Location/distribution*
Check lesion for generalized/ localized, body region, pat- terns, or discrete/confluent.

UNEXPECTED: See table on pp. 40-43.

Primary Skin Lesions

DESCRIPTION	EXAMPLES

Macule

Flat, circumscribed area that is a change in skin color; <1 cm in diameter

Freckles, flat moles (nevi), petechiae, measles, scarlet fever

Measles. (From Heinz F. Eichenwald, MD, Bob Craig; Public Health Image Library, Centers for Disease Control and Prevention.)

Papule

Elevated, firm, circumscribed area <1 cm in diameter

Wart (verruca), elevated moles, lichen planus

Lichen planus. (From Weston WL, et al: Color textbook of pediatric dermatology, ed 4, St Louis, 2007, Mosby.)

Patch

Flat, nonpalpable, irregular-shaped macule >1 cm in diameter

Vitiligo, port-wine stains, Mongolian spots, café-au-lait spots

Vitiligo. (From Brian Hill, New Zealand; PHIL, CDC.)

Primary Skin Lesions—cont'd

DESCRIPTION	EXAMPLES

Plaque

Elevated, firm, and rough lesion with flat-top surface >1 cm in diameter

Psoriasis, seborrheic and actinic keratosis

Psoriasis. (From Richard S. Hibbets; PHIL, CDC.)

Wheal

Elevated irregular-shaped area of cutaneous edema; solid, transient; variable diameter

Insect bites, urticaria, allergic reaction

Wheal. (From Dr. Frank Perlman, M.A. Parsons; PHIL, CDC.)

Nodule

Elevated, firm, circumscribed lesion; deeper in dermis than a papule; 1-2 cm in diameter

Erythema nodosum, lipomas

Hypertrophic nodule. (From Goldman MP, Fitzpatrick RE: Cutaneous laser surgery: the art and science of selective photothermolysis, St Louis, 1994, Mosby.)

Continued

DESCRIPTION	EXAMPLES

Tumor

Elevated and solid lesion; may or may not be clearly demarcated; deeper in dermis; >2 cm in diameter

Neoplasms, benign tumor, lipoma, hemangioma

Lipoma. (From Lemmi FO, Lemmi CAE: Physical assessment findings CD-ROM, Philadelphia, 2000, Saunders.)

Vesicle

Elevated, circumscribed, superficial, not into dermis; filled with serous fluid; <1 cm in diameter

Varicella (chickenpox), herpes zoster (shingles)

Vesicles caused by varicella. (From Dr. John Noble, Jr.; PHIL, CDC.)

Bulla

Vesicle >1 cm in diameter

Blister, pemphigus vulgaris

Blister. (From Weston et al, 2007.)

SKIN, HAIR, AND NAILS

Primary Skin Lesions—cont'd

| DESCRIPTION | EXAMPLES |

Pustule

Elevated, superficial lesion; similar to a vesicle but filled with purulent fluid

Impetigo, acne

Acne. (From Ferri, FF: Ferri's Color Atlas and Text of Clinical Medicine, Philadelphia, 2009, Saunders.)

Cyst

Elevated, circumscribed, encapsulated lesion; in dermis or subcutaneous layer; filled with liquid or semisolid material

Sebaceous cyst, cystic acne

Sebaceous cyst. (From Dr. Gavin Hart; PHIL, CDC.)

Telangiectasia

Fine, irregular red lines produced by capillary dilation

Telangiectasia in rosacea

Telangiectasia. (From Lemmi and Lemmi, 2000.)

TECHNIQUE	FINDINGS

Hair
Inspect hair over entire body

- *Color*

EXPECTED: Light blond to black and gray, with alterations caused by rinses, dyes, and permanents.

- *Distribution/quantity*

EXPECTED: Hair present on scalp, lower face, neck, nares, ears, chest, axillae, back and shoulders, arms, legs, pubic area, and around nipples. Scalp hair loss in adult men, adrenal androgenic female-pattern alopecia in adult women.

UNEXPECTED: Localized or generalized hair loss, inflammation, or scarring. Broken/absent hair shafts. Hirsutism in women.

Palpate for texture

EXPECTED: Coarse or fine, curly or straight, shiny, smooth, and resilient. Fine vellus covering body; coarse terminal hair on scalp, on pubis, on axillary areas, and in male beard.

UNEXPECTED: Dryness and brittleness.

Nails
Inspect nails

- *Color*

EXPECTED: Variations of pink with varying opacity. Pigment deposits in persons with dark skin. White spots.

UNEXPECTED: Yellow or green-black discoloration. Diffuse darkening. Pigment deposits in persons with light skin. Longitudinal red, brown, or white streaks or white bands. White, yellow, or green tinge. Blue nail beds. Blue-black discoloration.

TECHNIQUE	FINDINGS
• *Length/configuration/ symmetry*	EXPECTED: Varying shape, smooth and flat/slightly convex, with edges smooth and rounded. UNEXPECTED: Jagged, broken, or bitten edges or cuticles. Peeling. Absence of nail.
• *Cleanliness*	EXPECTED: Clean and neat. UNEXPECTED: Unkempt.
• *Ridging and beading*	EXPECTED: Longitudinal ridging and beading. UNEXPECTED: Longitudinal ridging and grooving with lichen planus. Transverse grooving, rippling, and depressions. Pitting.

Palpate nail plate

| • *Texture/firmness/thickness/ uniformity* | EXPECTED: Hard and smooth with uniform thickness. UNEXPECTED: Thickening or thinning. |
| • *Adherence to nail bed* Gently squeeze between thumb and finger. | EXPECTED: Firmness. UNEXPECTED: Separation. Boggy nail base. |

Measure nail base angle

| Inspect fingers when patient places dorsal surfaces of fingertips together. | EXPECTED: 160-degree angle. UNEXPECTED: Clubbing. |

Expected finding. (From Spicknall KE, et al: Clubbing: An update on diagnosis, differential diagnosis, pathophysiology, and clinical relevance, J Am Acad Dermatol 1020-1028, 2005.)

Clubbing. (From Spicknall KE, et al: Clubbing: An update on diagnosis, differential diagnosis, pathophysiology, and clinical relevance, J Am Acad Dermatol 1020-1028, 2005.)

Inspect and palpate proximal and lateral nail folds

UNEXPECTED: Redness, swelling, pus, warts, cysts, tumors, and pain.

AIDS TO DIFFERENTIAL DIAGNOSIS

SUBJECTIVE DATA	OBJECTIVE DATA

Eczematous Dermatitis

Itching may or may not be present; those with atopic dermatitis often report allergy history (allergic rhinitis, asthma).

Acute: erythematous, pruritic, weeping vesicles; subacute: erythema and scaling; chronic: thick, lichenified, pruritic plaques. Atopic dermatitis: during childhood, lesions involve flexures, the nape, and the dorsal aspects of the limbs. In adolescence and adulthood, lichenified plaques affect the flexures, head, and neck.

Folliculitis

Acute onset of papules and pustules associated with pruritus or mild discomfort; may have pain with deep folliculitis.

Primary lesion is a small pustule 1-2 cm in diameter that is located over a pilosebaceous orifice and may be perforated by a hair. Pustule may be surrounded by inflammation or nodular lesions. After the pustule ruptures, a crust forms.

Tinea (Dermatophytosis)

Pruritus.

Papular, pustular, vesicular, erythematous, or scaling lesions. Possible secondary bacterial infection. Hyphae on microscopic examination of skin scraping with KOH solution.

Rosacea

Common triggers: sun, cold weather, sudden emotion, hot beverages, spicy foods, and alcohol.

Telangiectasia, erythema, papules, and pustules particularly in the central area of the face; rhino-phyma may occur.

Herpes Zoster (Shingles)

Pain, itching, or burning usually precedes eruption by 4-5 days.

Red, swollen plaques or vesicles along a single dermatome.

SUBJECTIVE DATA	OBJECTIVE DATA
Basal Cell Carcinoma	
Persistent sore or lesions that have not healed; crusting; itching.	Shiny nodule that is pearly or translucent; may be pink, red, white, tan, black, or brown growth with a slightly elevated rolled border and a crusted indentation in the center.
Squamous Cell Carcinoma	
Persistent sore or lesion that has not healed or that has grown in size; crusting and/ or bleeding.	Elevated growth with a central depression, wartlike growth; scaly red patch with irregular borders; open sore.
Malignant Melanoma	
New mole or preexisting mole that has changed or is changing; history of melanoma, dysplastic or atypical nevi; family history of melanoma.	Characteristic asymmetry, irregular borders, variegated colors, and is growing or >6 mm (see ABCDs of Melanoma on pp. 49-50).
Hirsutism	
Growth of terminal hair in women in the male distribution pattern on the face, body, and pubic areas.	Presence of thick, dark terminal hairs in androgen-sensitive sites: face, chest, areola, external genitalia, upper and lower back, buttock, inner thigh, linea.
Paronychia	
Acute: history of nail trauma or manipulation; acute onset. Chronic: history of repeated exposure to moisture, e.g., through hand-washing. Evolves slowly initially with tenderness and mild swelling.	Redness, swelling, tenderness at lateral and proximal nail folds. Possible purulent drainage under cuticle. Acute or chronic (with nail rippling).

SUBJECTIVE DATA	OBJECTIVE DATA
Onychomycosis	
Yellow, crumbling nail.	Distal nail plate turns yellow or white as hyperkeratotic debris accumulates, causing the nail to separate from the nail bed. Redness and swelling where nail pierces the lateral nail fold and grows into the dermis.

PEDIATRIC VARIATIONS

EXAMINATION

TECHNIQUE	FINDINGS
Skin	
Inspect hands and feet of newborns for skin creases	
	EXPECTED: Number of creases is indication of maturity of newborn; the older the gestational age, the more creases. UNEXPECTED: Single transverse crease across palm often seen in infants with Down syndrome.

AIDS TO DIFFERENTIAL DIAGNOSIS

SUBJECTIVE DATA	OBJECTIVE DATA
Seborrheic Dermatitis	
Thick, greasy scalp scales or body rash.	Thick, yellow, adherent crusted scalp, ear, or neck lesions.
Impetigo	
Lesion, typically on the face, that itches and burns.	Honey-colored crusted or ruptured vesicles.
Miliaria ("Prickly Heat")	
Parent reports rash noted while undressing infant.	Irregular, red, macular rash on covered areas.

SUBJECTIVE DATA	OBJECTIVE DATA
Chickenpox (Varicella)	
Fever, headache, sore throat, malaise.	Pruritic maculopapular skin eruption that becomes vesicular in a matter of hours.
German Measles (Rubella)	
Fever, coryza, sore throat, cough.	Koplik spots on buccal mucosa; generalized light pink to red maculopapular rash.

Sample Documentation

Objective

Skin: Dark pink maculopapular lesions on face, torso, extremities; large urticarial wheal on right cheek. No excoriation or secondary infection. Turgor resilient. Skin uniformly warm and dry. No edema.

Hair: Curly, black, thick with female distribution pattern. Texture coarse.

Nails: Opaque, short, well-groomed, uniform, and without deformities. Nail bed pink. Nail base angle 160 degrees. No redness, exudates, or swelling in surrounding folds and no tenderness to palpation.

The ABCDs of Melanoma

Characteristics that should alert you to the possibility of malignant melanoma:

A Asymmetry of lesion: Half of a mole or birthmark does not match the other.

B Borders: Edges are irregular, ragged, notched, or blurred. Pigment may be streaming from the border.

C Color: The color is not the same all over and may have differing shades of brown or black, sometimes with patches of red, white, or blue.

D Diameter: The diameter is larger than 6 mm (about the size of a pencil eraser) or is growing larger.

E Evolution: Changes seen in existing pigmented lesions, particularly in a nonuniform, asymmetric manner.

Asymmetry   Color

Border   Diameter

Melanoma. (Reproduced with permission from the American Academy of Dermatology, 2010. All rights reserved.)

Lymphatic System

Equipment

- Centimeter ruler
- Skin-marking pencil

EXAMINATION

The lymphatic system is examined by inspection and palpation, region by region, during the examination of other body systems, and by palpating the spleen. If enlarged nodes are found, inspect regions drained by nodes for infection or malignancy and examine other regions for enlargement.

Lymph Nodes Most Accessible to Inspection and Palpation

The more superficial the node, the more accessible it is to your palpation.

"Necklace" of Nodes
Parotid and retropharyngeal (tonsillar)
Submandibular
Submental
Sublingual (facial)
Superficial anterior cervical
Superficial posterior cervical
Preauricular and postauricular

Occipital
Supraclavicular

Arms
Axillary
Epitrochlear (cubital)

Legs
Superficial superior inguinal
Superficial inferior inguinal
Occasionally, popliteal

TECHNIQUE	FINDINGS

Head and Neck
Inspect for visible nodes
Ask if patient is aware of any lumps.

UNEXPECTED: Edema, erythema, red streaks, or lesions.

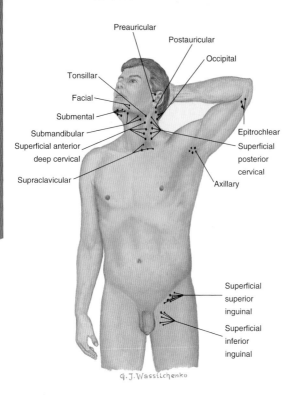

Preauricular
Postauricular
Occipital
Tonsillar
Facial
Submental
Submandibular
Superficial anterior
deep cervical
Supraclavicular
Epitrochlear
Superficial
posterior
cervical
Axillary
Superficial
superior
inguinal
Superficial
inferior
inguinal

G.J. Wassilchenko

TECHNIQUE

FINDINGS

Palpate superficial nodes; note size, consistency, mobility, tenderness, warmth

Bend patient's head slightly forward or to side. Palpate gently with pads of second, third, fourth fingers.

- *Occipital nodes at base of skull*
- *Postauricular nodes over mastoid process*
- *Preauricular nodes in front of ears*
- *Parotid and retropharyngeal nodes at angle of mandible*
- *Submandibular nodes between angle and tip of mandible*
- *Submental nodes behind tip of mandible*

EXPECTED: Nodes not palpable.
UNEXPECTED: Enlarged, tender, red or discolored, fixed, matted, inflamed, or warm nodes; increased vascularity.

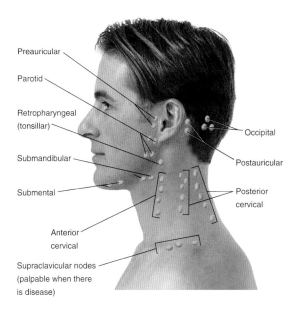

Preauricular

Parotid

Retropharyngeal
(tonsillar)

Occipital

Submandibular

Postauricular

Submental

Posterior
cervical

Anterior
cervical

Supraclavicular nodes
(palpable when there
is disease)

Neck

- *Superficial cervical nodes at sternocleidomastoid*
- *Posterior cervical nodes along anterior border of trapezius*
- *Deep cervical nodes along anterior border of trapezius*
- *Supraclavicular areas* Hook fingers over clavicle and rotate over supraclavicular fossa while patient turns head toward same side and raises shoulder.

EXPECTED: Nodes not palpable.
UNEXPECTED: Enlarged, tender, red or discolored, fixed, matted, inflamed, or warm nodes; increased vascularity.

UNEXPECTED: Detection of Virchow nodes.
Note: A palpable supraclavicular node should always make you suspect the probability of a malignancy.

TECHNIQUE	FINDINGS

Axillae

Inspect for visible nodes

Ask if patient is aware of any lumps.

UNEXPECTED: Edema, erythema, red streaks, or lesions.

Palpate superficial nodes for size, consistency, mobility, tenderness, warmth

Using firm, deliberate, gentle touch, rotate fingertips and palm. Attempt to glide fingers beneath nodes.

Axillary Nodes

Support patient's forearm and bring palm of examining hand flat into axilla. With palmar surface of fingers, reach deep into hollow, pushing firmly upward, then bring fingers down, rotating your fingers and gently rolling soft tissue against chest wall and axilla. Explore apex, medial, lateral aspects along rib cage; lateral aspects along upper surface of arm; and anterior and posterior walls of axilla. Repeat mirror image of this maneuver for the other axilla.

EXPECTED: Nodes not palpable. UNEXPECTED: Enlarged, tender, red or discolored, fixed, matted, inflamed, or warm nodes; increased vascularity.

Other Lymph Nodes

Inspect visible nodes

Ask if patient is aware of any lumps.

UNEXPECTED: Edema, erythema, red streaks, or lesions.

TECHNIQUE	FINDINGS

Palpate superficial nodes for size, consistency, mobility, tenderness, warmth

Systematically palpate other areas, moving hand in circular fashion, probing without pressing hard.

EXPECTED: Nodes not palpable.
UNEXPECTED: Enlarged, tender, red or discolored, fixed, matted, inflamed, or warm nodes; increased vascularity.

- *Epitrochlear nodes*
  Support elbow in one hand while exploring with other. Palpate that groove between the triceps and biceps muscle with your fingers using a circular motion.

- *Inguinal area*
  Have patient lie supine with knee slightly flexed. The superior superficial inguinal (femoral) nodes are close to the surface over the inguinal canals. The inferior superficial inguinal nodes lie deeper in the groin.

- *Popliteal nodes*
  Relax the posterior popliteal fossa by flexing the knee. Wrap your hand around the knee and palpate the fossa with your fingers.

AIDS TO DIFFERENTIAL DIAGNOSIS

SUBJECTIVE DATA	OBJECTIVE DATA
Acute Lymphangitis	
Pain, malaise, illness, possibly fever.	Red streak (tracing of fine lines) may follow course of lymphatic collecting duct. Inflamed area indurated and palpable to gentle touch. Related infection possible distally, particularly interdigitally.
Non-Hodgkin Lymphoma	
Painless enlarged lymph node(s); fever, weight loss, night sweats, abdominal pain or fullness.	Nodes may be localized in the posterior cervical triangle or may become matted, crossing into the anterior triangle nodes; usually well defined and solid.
Hodgkin Lymphoma	
Painless progressive enlargement of cervical lymph nodes. Generally asymmetric.	Nodes sometimes matted and generally very firm, almost rubbery.
Epstein-Barr Virus; Mononucleosis	
Pharyngitis, fever, fatigue, malaise.	Commonly splenomegaly and/or rash. Palpable nodes generalized but more commonly in anterior and posterior cervical chains. Nodes vary in firmness, are generally discrete, are occasionally tender.
Roseola Infantum (Human Herpesvirus 6)	
Fever: usually high grade and persistent over 3 to 4 days; sometimes associated with a mild respiratory illness.	Discrete and nontender nodes in the occipital and postauricular chains.

SUBJECTIVE DATA	OBJECTIVE DATA
Herpes Simplex	
Burning, itching lesions; enlarged lymph nodes.	Discrete labial and gingival ulcers, high fever, enlargement of anterior cervical and submandibular nodes. Nodes tend to be firm, quite discrete, movable, tender.
Human Immunodeficiency Virus/Acquired Immunodeficiency Syndrome (HIV/AIDS)	
Severe fatigue, malaise, weakness, persistent diarrhea; arthralgias.	Lymphadenopathy, fever, unexplained weight loss.

Terms

Conditions
Lymphadenopathy (adenopathy)—enlarged lymph node(s)
Lymphadenitis—inflamed and enlarged lymph node(s)
Lymphangitis—inflammation of the lymphatics that drain an area of infection; tender erythematous streaks extend proximally from the infected area; regional nodes may also be tender
Lymphedema—edematous swelling caused by excess accumulation of lymph fluid in tissues caused by inadequate lymph drainage
Lymphangioma—congenital malformation of dilated lymphatics

Nodes
Shotty—small nontender nodes that feel like BBs or buckshot under the skin
Fluctuant—wavelike motion that is felt when the node is palpated
Matted—group of nodes that feel connected and seem to move as a unit

Some Conditions That Simulate Lymph Node Enlargement

Lymphangioma
Hemangioma (tends to feel spongy; appears reddish blue, depending on size and extent of angiomatous involvement)
Branchial cleft cyst (sometimes accompanied by tiny orifice in neck on line extending to ear)
Thyroglossal duct cyst
Laryngocele
Esophageal diverticulum
Thyroid goiter
Graves disease
Hashimoto thyroiditis
Parotid swelling (e.g., from mumps or tumor)

Differential Diagnosis Lymphedema or Edema?

- Both can be either pitting or nonpitting.
- Except in early stages, lymphedema does not resolve with elevation of the affected area.
- Edema secondary to increased capillary filtration (e.g., chronic venous insufficiency) usually improves.
- Diuretics do not help lymphedema. They may help edema from other causes.
- Be aware that some patients may have both edema and lymphedema.

PEDIATRIC VARIATIONS

EXAMINATION

TECHNIQUE	FINDINGS

Head and Neck
Palpate superficial nodes

- *Occipital nodes at base of skull*
- *Postauricular nodes over mastoid process*

EXPECTED: In children, small, firm, discrete, nontender, nonmovable nodes in occipital, postauricular chains.

Other Lymph Nodes
Palpate superficial nodes

- *Inguinal and popliteal areas*

EXPECTED: In children, small, firm, discrete nodes; nontender, movable in inguinal chain.

Sample Documentation

Subjective. A 25-year-old woman reports difficulty swallowing and sore throat for 3 days, now subsiding, and fever up to 38°C (100.5°F) for 2 days. Has been using acetaminophen and throat lozenges for pain relief.

Objective. No visible enlargement of lymph nodes in any area. Enlarged node (2 cm in diameter) palpated in left posterior cervical triangle; firm, nontender, movable, no overlying warmth, erythema, or edema. A few shotty nodes palpated in posterior cervical triangles bilaterally and in femoral chains bilaterally.

CHAPTER

7   **Head and Neck**

Equipment

- Tape measure
- Cup of water
- Stethoscope
- Transilluminator

EXAMINATION

Ask patient to sit.

TECHNIQUE	FINDINGS

Head and Face
Observe head position

EXPECTED: Upright, midline, still.
UNEXPECTED: Tilted, horizontal jerking or bobbing, tics, nodding.

Inspect facial features

- *Shape*
  Observe eyelids, eyebrows, palpebral fissures, nasolabial folds, mouth at rest, during movement, with expression.

EXPECTED: Variations according to race, sex, age, body build.
UNEXPECTED: Change in shape. Unusual features: edema, puffiness, coarsened features, prominent eyes, hirsutism, lack of expression, excessive perspiration, pallor, or pigmentation variations.

- *Symmetry*
  Note if asymmetry affects all features of one side or a portion of face.

EXPECTED: Slight asymmetry.
UNEXPECTED: Facial nerve weakness or paralysis, or problem with peripheral trigeminal nerve.

TECHNIQUE	FINDINGS
Inspect skull and scalp	
• *Size/shape/symmetry* • *Scalp condition* • *Systematically part hair from frontal to occipital region.*	EXPECTED: Symmetric. UNEXPECTED: Lesions, scabs, tenderness, parasites, nits, scaliness.
• *Hair pattern* Pay special attention to areas behind ears, at hairline, at crown.	EXPECTED: Bitemporal recession or balding over crown in men. UNEXPECTED: Random areas of alopecia or alopecia totalis.
Palpate head and scalp	
• *Symmetry* Palpate in gentle, rotary motion from front to back.	EXPECTED: Symmetric and smooth with bones indistinguishable. Ridge of sagittal fissure occasionally palpable. UNEXPECTED: Indentations or depressions.
Palpate hair	
• *Texture/color distribution*	EXPECTED: Smooth, symmetrically distributed. UNEXPECTED: Splitting or cracked ends. Coarse, dry, or brittle. Fine and silky.
Palpate temporal arteries Note course of arteries.	UNEXPECTED: Thickening, hardness, or tenderness.

Auscultate temporal arteries and over skull and eyes

EXPECTED: No bruits.

TECHNIQUE	FINDINGS

Inspect salivary glands

- *Symmetry/size*
  Palpate if asymmetry noted.
  Have patient open mouth
  and press on salivary duct
  to attempt to express
  material.

UNEXPECTED: Asymmetry or enlargement. Tenderness. Discrete
nodule.

Neck

Inspect neck

- *Symmetry*
  Inspect in usual position, in
  slight hyperextension, and
  during swallowing. Look for
  landmarks of anterior and
  posterior triangles.

EXPECTED: Bilateral symmetry of
sternocleidomastoid and trapezius muscles.
UNEXPECTED: Asymmetry, torticol-
lis, webbing, excessive posterior
skinfolds, unusually short neck,
distention of jugular vein;
prominence of carotid arteries or
edema.

- *Trachea*
  Inspect in usual position,
  in slight hyperextension,
  and while patient swallows.

EXPECTED: Midline placement.
UNEXPECTED: Masses.

Evaluate range of motion

Have patient flex, extend,
rotate, laterally turn head and
neck.

EXPECTED: Smooth.
UNEXPECTED: Pain, dizziness, or
limitation of motion.

Palpate neck

- *Trachea*
  Place thumb on each side
  of trachea in lower portion
  of neck, and compare space
  between trachea and
  sternocleidomastoid on
  each side.

EXPECTED: Midline position.
UNEXPECTED: Deviation to right
or left.

TECHNIQUE   FINDINGS

- *Hyoid bone/thyroid and cricoid cartilages*
  Have patient swallow.
- *Cartilaginous rings of trachea*
  Have patient swallow.

EXPECTED: Smooth. Moves during swallowing.
UNEXPECTED: Tender.
EXPECTED: Distinct.
UNEXPECTED: Tender.

- *Tracheal tug*
  With neck extended, palpate for movement with index finger and thumb on each side of trachea below thyroid isthmus.

UNEXPECTED: Tug synchronous with pulse.

Palpate lymph nodes

- *Size/consistency, mobility/ condition*

UNEXPECTED: Enlarged, matted, tender, fixed, warm.

Palpate thyroid gland

- *Symmetry*
  Observe from frontal and lateral positions while patient hyperextends neck. Then observe as patient sips water while neck is hyperextended.

UNEXPECTED: Asymmetry. En-larged and visible thyroid gland.

HEAD AND NECK

TECHNIQUE	FINDINGS
• *Size/shape/configuration/ consistency* Stand either facing or behind patient. Have patient hold head slightly forward and tipped toward side being examined. Lightly palpate isthmus and lateral lobes. Give water to patient to facilitate swallowing. From the front, examine the left lobe by sitting on the left side of the patient and pressing the trachea to the left with the left thumb. Place the first three fingers in the thyroid bed just medial to the sternocleidomastoid. Keep your fingers still while the patient again swallows, thereby moving the gland beneath your fingers. Repeat on the right side. If gland is enlarged, auscultate for vascular sounds with stethoscope bell.	EXPECTED: Lobes small and smooth. Gland rises freely with swallowing. Right lobe as much as 25% larger than left. Tissue firm and pliable. UNEXPECTED: Enlarged, tender nodules (smooth or irregular, soft or hard); coarse tissue; gritty sensation. UNEXPECTED: Bruit.

AIDS TO DIFFERENTIAL DIAGNOSIS

SUBJECTIVE DATA | OBJECTIVE DATA

Myxedema

Cognitive impairment, slowed mentation, poor concentration, decreased short-term memory, social withdrawal, psychomotor retardation, depressed mood, and apathy.

Dull, puffy, yellow skin. Coarse, sparse hair. Temporal loss of eyebrows. Periorbital edema. Prominent tongue. Hypothyroidism (see table on p. 68).

Graves Disease

Symptoms of hyperthyroidism, palpitations, heat intolerance, weight loss, fatigue, increased appetite, tachycardia.

Diffuse thyroid enlargement, hyperthyroidism. Various pathologic conditions—ophthalmologic (prominent eyes, lid retraction, staring or startled expression), dermatologic (fine and moist skin, fine hair), musculoskeletal (muscle weakness), cardiac (tachycardia) (see table on p. 68).

HEAD AND NECK

Headaches

Headaches are one of the most common concerns and probably one of the most self-medicated. They are not always benign. A history of insistent headache that is severe and recurrent must be given attention. Sometimes the underlying cause is life-threatening, such as a brain tumor. Sometimes it affects daily activities. The patient's history is fully as important as the physical examination in getting at the root of a headache. Various kinds of headaches can be compared as follows:

CHARAC-TERISTIC	CLASSIC MIGRAINE	MEDICATION REBOUND	CLUSTER	HYPERTEN-SIVE	MUSCULAR TENSION	TEMPORAL ARTERITIS	SPACE-OCCUPYING LESION
Age at onset	Childhood		Adulthood	Adulthood	Adulthood	Older adulthood	Any
Location	Unilateral or generalized	Holocranial or diffuse	Unilateral	Bilateral or occipital	Unilateral or bilateral	Unilateral or bilateral	Localized
Duration	Hours to days	Hours	½ to 2 hours	Hours	Hours to days	Hours to days	Rapidly increasing frequency
Time of onset	Morning or night	Predictably begins within hours to days of the last dose of the medication	Night	Morning	Anytime, commonly in afternoon or evening	Anytime	Awakening from sleep
Quality of pain	Pulsating or throbbing	Dull or throbbing	Intense burning, boring, searing, knifelike	Throbbing	Bandlike, constricting	Throbbing	

Prodromal event	Vague neurologic changes, personality change, fluid retention, appetite loss / Well-defined neurologic event, scotoma, aphasia, hemianopsia, aura	Daily analgesic use	Personality changes, sleep disturbances	None	None	None	Aggravated by coughing or bending forward
Precipitating event	Menstrual period, missing meals, birth control pills, letdown after stress	Abrupt discontinuation of analgesics	Alcohol consumption	None	Stress, anger, bruxism	None	Develops in temporal relation to the neoplasm
Frequency	Twice a week	Gradual increase in headache frequency to daily	Several times nightly for several nights, then none	Daily	Daily	Daily	Progressive
Sex predilection	Females	Females	Males	Equal	Equal	Equal	Equal
Other symptoms	Nausea, vomiting	Alternate or preventive medications fail to control the headache	Increased lacrimation, nasal discharge	Generally remits as day progresses	None	None	Vomiting, confusion, abnormal neurologic findings, gait abnormality, papilledema, nystagmus

HEAD AND NECK

Hyperthyroidism Versus Hypothyroidism

SYSTEM OR STRUCTURE AFFECTED	HYPERTHYROIDISM	HYPOTHYROIDISM
Constitutional		
Temperature preference	Cool climate	Warm climate
Weight	Loss	Gain
Emotional state	Nervous, easily irritated, highly energetic	Lethargic, complacent, uninterested
Hair	Fine, with hair loss; failure to hold permanent wave	Coarse, with tendency to break
Skin	Warm, fine, hyperpigmentation at pressure points	Coarse, scaling, dry
Fingernails	Thin, with tendency to break; may show onycholysis	Thick
Eyes	Bilateral or unilateral proptosis, lid retraction, double vision	Puffiness in periorbital region
Neck	Goiter, change in shirt neck size, pain over thyroid	No goiter
Cardiac	Tachycardia, dysrhythmia, palpitations	No change noted
Gastrointestinal	Increased frequency of bowel movements; diarrhea rare	Constipation
Menstrual	Scant flow, amenorrhea	Menorrhagia
Neuromuscular	Increasing weakness, especially of proximal muscles	Lethargic but good muscular strength

PEDIATRIC VARIATIONS

EXAMINATION

TECHNIQUE	FINDINGS

Head and Face

Palpate head and scalp

- *Symmetry*
  In infants, transilluminate skull

  EXPECTED: An infant's head circumference is 2 cm greater than chest circumference up to the age of 2 yr.
  UNEXPECTED: Ring of light >2 cm with transillumination.

TECHNIQUE	FINDINGS

- *Skull condition*

EXPECTED: In infants, posterior fontanel closed at 2 mo; anterior fontanel closed at 12-15 mo.
UNEXPECTED: Tenderness or depressions; sunken areas; swelling, bulging, or depressed fontanels.

- *Scalp*

EXPECTED: Free movement.
UNEXPECTED: Fixation of scalp, bulging either on one side or crossing midline of scalp.

Percuss skull

EXPECTED: Macewen sign, percussion near junction of frontal, temporal, and parietal bones producing a stronger resonant sound, is physiologic when fontanels are open.
UNEXPECTED: Macewen sign may indicate hydrocephalus, brain abscess, or increased intracranial pressure after fontanel closure.

Auscultate temporal arteries and over skull and eyes

EXPECTED: Bruits are common in children up to age 5 yr.

Neck

Palpate thyroid gland

- *Symmetry*

EXPECTED: In children, thyroid gland may be palpable.
UNEXPECTED: Tenderness.

HEAD AND NECK

Sample Documentation

Head. Held erect and midline. Skull normocephalic, symmetric, smooth without deformities. Facial features symmetric. Salivary glands not inflamed or tender. Temporal artery pulsations visible bilaterally, soft and nontender to palpation. No bruits.

Neck. Trachea midline. No jugular venous distention or carotid artery prominence. Thyroid palpable, firm, smooth, not enlarged. Thyroid and cartilages move with swallowing. No nodules or tenderness. No bruits. Full range of motion of neck without discomfort.

Eyes

Equipment

- Snellen chart or Lea cards, Landolt C or HOTV chart
- Eye cover, gauze, or opaque card
- Rosenbaum or Jaeger near-vision card
- Penlight
- Cotton wisp
- Ophthalmoscope

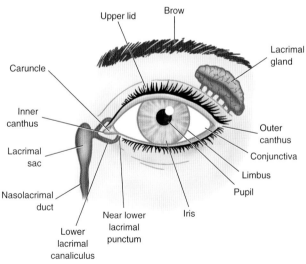

(Thompson JM, et al: Mosby's clinical nursing, ed 4, St Louis, 1997, Mosby.)

EYES

EXAMINATION

Ask patient to sit or stand.

TECHNIQUE   FINDINGS

Visual Testing
Measure visual acuity in each eye separately

- *Distance vision*
  Use Snellen chart, Landolt
  C, or HOTV chart. If testing
  with and without corrective
  lenses, test without lenses
  first and record readings
  separately.

- *Near vision*
  Use near-vision card.

- *Peripheral vision*
  Test nasal, temporal, superior,
  inferior fields by moving your
  finger into field from outside.

EXPECTED: Vision 20/20 with
or without lenses with near
and far vision in each eye.
UNEXPECTED: Myopia, amblyo-
pia, or presbyopia.

EXPECTED: Vision 20/20.
UNEXPECTED: Limited fields
of vision temporally, 50
degrees superiorly, 70 degrees
inferiorly.

External Examination
Inspect eyebrows

- *Size/extension*

- *Hair texture*

EXPECTED: Unusually thin if
plucked.
UNEXPECTED: Ending short of
temporal canthus.
UNEXPECTED: Coarse.

TECHNIQUE	FINDINGS

Inspect orbital area

UNEXPECTED: Edema, puffiness not related to aging, or sagging tissue below orbit. Xanthelasma.

Inspect eyelids

- *Eyelid position*

  UNEXPECTED: Ectropion or entropion.

- *Ability to open wide and close completely*
  Examine with eyes lightly closed, closed tightly, open wide.

  EXPECTED: Superior eyelid covering a portion of iris when open.
  UNEXPECTED: Fasciculations when lightly closed. Ptosis. Lagophthalmos.

- *Eyelid margin*

  UNEXPECTED: Flakiness, redness, or swelling. Hordeola.

- *Eyelashes*

  EXPECTED: Present on both lids. Turned outward.

Palpate eyelids

UNEXPECTED: Nodules.

Palpate eye

EXPECTED: Can be gently pushed into orbit without discomfort.
UNEXPECTED: Firm and resists palpation.

Pull down lower lids and inspect conjunctivae and sclerae

- *Color*
  Inspect upper tarsal conjunctivae only if presence of foreign body is suspected.

  EXPECTED: Conjunctivae clear and inapparent. Sclerae white and visible above irides only when eyelids are wide open.
  UNEXPECTED: Conjunctivae with erythema. Sclerae yellow or green. Sclerae with dark, rust-colored pigment anterior to insertion of medial rectus muscle.

EYES

TECHNIQUE	FINDINGS
• *Appearance*	UNEXPECTED: Exudate. Pterygium. Corneal arcus senilis or opacities.

Inspect lacrimal gland region

• *Lacrimal gland puncta* Palpate lower orbital rim near inner canthus. If temporal aspect of upper lid feels full, evert lid and inspect gland.	EXPECTED: Slight elevations with central depression on both upper and lower lid margins. UNEXPECTED: Enlarged glands. Dry eyes.

Test corneal sensitivity

Touch wisp of cotton to cornea.	EXPECTED: Bilateral blink reflex.

Inspect external eyes

• *Corneal clarity* Shine light tangentially on cornea.	UNEXPECTED: Blood vessels present.
• *Irides*	EXPECTED: Clearly visible pattern. Similar color.
• *Pupillary size/shape*	EXPECTED: Round, regular, equal in size. UNEXPECTED: Miosis, mydriasis, anisocoria, or coloboma.
• *Pupillary response to light*	EXPECTED: Constricting with consensual response of opposite pupil.
• *Pupillary accommodation*	EXPECTED: Constricting when pupils focus on near object or dilating when focus changes from near to distant object.
• *Afferent pupillary testing*	EXPECTED: The pupil toward which the light is moving dilates and then constricts as the light shines onto it. UNEXPECTED: The pupil continues to dilate when the light shines into it.

TECHNIQUE   FINDINGS

Extraocular Eye Muscles
Evaluate muscle balance and movement of eyes

- *Six cardinal fields of gaze*
  Hold patient's chin and ask
  patient to watch finger or
  penlight.

EXPECTED: A few horizontal
nystagmic beats. Smooth,
full, coordinated movement
of eyes.
UNEXPECTED: Sustained or
jerking nystagmus. Exposure
of sclera from lid lag.
Inability of eye to move in all
directions.

Superior rectus, CN III — Inferior oblique, CN III — Inferior oblique, CN III — Superior rectus, CN III — Medial rectus, CN III — Lateral rectus, CN VI — Lateral rectus, CN VI — Inferior rectus, CN III — Superior oblique, CN IV — Superior oblique, CN IV — Inferior rectus, CN III

- *Corneal light reflex*
  Direct light at nasal bridge
  from 30 cm (12 inches). Have
  patient look at nearby object.

EXPECTED: Light reflected
symmetrically from both eyes.

- *Cover-uncover test*
  Perform if imbalance found
  with corneal light reflex test.
  Have patient stare ahead at
  near, fixed object. Cover one
  eye and observe the other;
  remove cover and observe
  uncovered eye. Repeat with
  other eye.

UNEXPECTED: Movement of
covered or uncovered eye.

EYES

TECHNIQUE	FINDINGS

Ophthalmoscopic Examination
Inspect internal eye

- *Lens clarity*

UNEXPECTED: Cloudiness or opacity. Shallow chamber. If observed, avoid mydriatics.

- *Anterior chamber*
  Shine focused light tangentially at limbus. Note illumination of iris nasally.

- *Use ophthalmoscope*
  With patient looking at distant object, direct light at pupil from about 30 cm (12 inches). Move toward patient, observing:
- *Red reflex*
- *Fundus*

UNEXPECTED: Opacities.
EXPECTED: Yellow or pink background, depending on race. Possible crescents or dots of pigment at disc margin, usually temporally.
UNEXPECTED: Discrete areas of pigmentation away from disc. Lesions. Drusen bodies. Hemorrhages.

TECHNIQUE

FINDINGS

- *Blood vessel characteristics* Follow blood vessels distally in each quadrant, noting crossings of arterioles and venules.

EXPECTED: Possible venous pulsations (should be documented). Arteriole/venule ratio 3:5 or 2:3.
UNEXPECTED: Nicking, tortuosity.

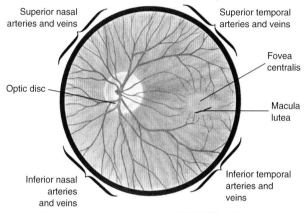

Superior nasal arteries and veins

Superior temporal arteries and veins

Fovea centralis

Optic disc

Macula lutea

Inferior nasal arteries and veins

Inferior temporal arteries and veins

- *Disc characteristics*

EXPECTED: Yellow to creamy pink, varying by race. Sharp, well-defined margin, especially in temporal region; 1.5-mm diameter.
UNEXPECTED: Myelinated nerve fibers. Papilledema. Glaucomatous cupping.

- *Macula densa characteristics* Ask patient to look directly at light.

EXPECTED: Yellow dot surrounded by deep pink.

EYES

EYES

AIDS TO DIFFERENTIAL DIAGNOSIS

SUBJECTIVE DATA	OBJECTIVE DATA

Strabismus (Paralytic and Nonparalytic)

Eyes cannot focus simultaneously. Can focus separately in nonparalytic type.

Eye movement on the cover-uncover test, strabismic eye will fixate on the object after the "straight" eye is covered.

Episcleritis

Acute onset of mild to moderate discomfort or photophobia. Painless injection and/or watery discharge.

Injection of the bulbar conjunctiva purplish elevation of a few millimeters.

Cataracts

Cloudy or blurry vision, faded colors; halo may appear around lights.

Opacity of lens, generally central, occasionally peripheral.

Diabetic Retinopathy (Background or Nonproliferative)

Initially asymptomatic. Blurred vision, distortion, or visual acuity loss in more advanced stages.

Dot hemorrhages, microaneurysms, hard exudates.

Diabetic Retinopathy (Proliferative)

Generally asymptomatic, floaters, blurred vision, or progressive visual acuity loss in advanced stages.

New vessel formation; extension out of the retina, hemorrhage.

PEDIATRIC VARIATIONS

EXAMINATION

TECHNIQUE	FINDINGS

Visual Testing

Measure visual acuity

- *Distance vision*
  Visual acuity is tested, when
  child is cooperative, with Lea
  cards, Landolt C, or HOTV
  chart, usually at about 3 years
  of age.

  EXPECTED: Infants should be able
  to focus on and track a face or
  light through 60 degrees. Age 3
  to 5 years: 20/40 or better. Age 6
  years: 20/30 or better.

Extraocular Eye Muscles

Evaluate muscle balance and movement of eyes

Evaluation of six cardinal fields of gaze is performed as with adults.
You may, however, need to hold child's head still.

Sample Documentation

Eyes. Near vision 20/40 in each eye uncorrected, corrected to 20/20
with glasses. Distant vision 20/20 by Snellen. Visual fields full by
confrontation. Extraocular movements intact and full, no nystagmus.
Corneal light reflex equal.

Lids and globes symmetric. No ptosis. Eyebrows full, no edema or
lesions evident.

Conjunctivae pink, sclerae white. No discharge evident. Cornea
clear, corneal reflex intact. Irides brown; pupils equal, round, reactive
to light and accommodation.

Ophthalmoscopic examination reveals red reflex. Discs cream
colored, borders well defined with temporal pigmentation in both
eyes. No venous pulsations evident at disc. Arteriole/venule ratio 3:5;
no nicking or crossing changes, hemorrhages, or exudates noted.
Maculae are yellow in each eye.

EYES

9 Ears, Nose, and Throat

Equipment

- Otoscope with pneumatic attachment
- Nasal speculum
- Tongue blades
- Tuning fork (approximate vocal frequencies between 512 Hz and 1024 Hz)
- Gauze
- Gloves
- Penlight, sinus transilluminator, or light from otoscope

EXAMINATION

Ask patient to sit.

TECHNIQUE	FINDINGS

Ears

Inspect auricles and mastoid area

Examine lateral and medial surfaces and surrounding tissue.

Helix
Triangular fossa
Antihelix
Concha
Antitragus
External auditory meatus
Tragus
Lobule

Auricle landmarks.

- *Size/shape/symmetry*

EXPECTED: Familial variations. Auricles of equal size and similar appearance. Darwin tubercle (congenital thickening along upper ridge of helix).

TECHNIQUE	FINDINGS
	UNEXPECTED: Unequal size or configuration. Cauliflower ear and other deformities.
• *Lesions*	UNEXPECTED: Moles, cysts or other lesions, nodules, or tophi (small whitish uric acid crystal deposition).
• *Color*	EXPECTED: Same color as facial skin.
	UNEXPECTED: Blueness, pallor, or excessive redness.
• *Position* Draw imaginary line between inner canthus of the eye and most prominent protuberance of occiput. Draw imaginary line perpendicular to first line and anterior to auricle.	EXPECTED: Top of auricle touching or above horizontal line. Auricle is in vertical position.
	UNEXPECTED: Auricle positioned below line (low-set); unequal alignment. Lateral posterior angle >10 degrees.
• *Preauricular area*	EXPECTED: Preauricular pits, skin tags, or smooth skin.
	UNEXPECTED: Openings in preauricular area, discharge.
• *External auditory canal*	EXPECTED: No discharge, no odor; canal walls pink.
	UNEXPECTED: Serous, bloody, or purulent discharge; foul smell.

Palpate auricles and mastoid area

	EXPECTED: Firm and mobile, readily recoils from folded position; no tenderness in postauricular or mastoid area.
	UNEXPECTED: Tenderness, swelling, nodules. Pain when pulling on lobule.

TECHNIQUE	FINDINGS
Inspect auditory canal with otoscope	
Using largest speculum that fits comfortably in the ear, slowly insert the otoscope speculum to a depth of 1 to 1½ cm (½ inch) inspecting the auditory canal from the meatus to the tympanic membrane.	EXPECTED: Minimal cerumen in varying color and texture. Uniformly pink canal. Hairs in outer third of canal. UNEXPECTED: Cerumen obscures tympanic membrane, odor, lesions, discharge, scaling, excessive redness, foreign body.
Inspect tympanic membrane	
• *Landmarks* Vary light direction to observe entire membrane and annulus.	EXPECTED: Visible landmarks (umbo, handle of malleus, light reflex). UNEXPECTED: Perforations, landmarks not visible.
• *Color*	EXPECTED: Translucent, pearly gray. UNEXPECTED: Amber, yellow, blue, deep red, chalky white, dull, white flecks, or dense white plaques; air bubbles or fluid level.

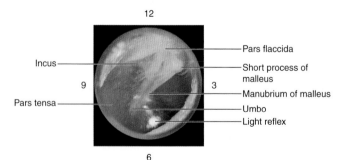

Tympanic membrane. (From Barkauskas et al, 2002.)

TECHNIQUE	FINDINGS
• *Contour*	EXPECTED: Slightly conical with concavity at umbo. UNEXPECTED: Bulging (more conical, usually with loss of bony landmarks and distorted light reflex) or retracted (more concave, usually with accentuated bony landmarks and distorted light reflex).
• *Mobility* Seal canal with speculum, and gently apply positive (squeeze bulb) and negative (release bulb) pressure with pneumatic attachment.	EXPECTED: Tympanic membrane moves in and out. UNEXPECTED: No movement of tympanic membrane.

Assess hearing

• *Questions asked during history*	EXPECTED: Responds to questions appropriately. UNEXPECTED: Excessive requests for repetition. Speech with monotonous tone and erratic volume.
• *Whispered voice* Have patient mask hearing in one ear by having patient gently occlude the nontested ear. Stand behind and to the side of patient at arm's length from the nontested ear and softly whisper combinations of three letters and numbers (e.g., 3, T, 9 or 5, M, 2). Ask patient to repeat what was heard. Use a different letter-number combination in other ear.	EXPECTED: Patient repeats numbers and letters correctly more than 50% of time. UNEXPECTED: Patient unable to repeat whispered words.

EARS, NOSE, AND THROAT

TECHNIQUE	FINDINGS

- *Weber test*
  Place base of vibrating tuning fork on midline vertex of head. To test patient's reliability, repeat with one ear occluded.

EXPECTED: Sound heard equally in both ears when ears are not occluded. Sound heard better in occluded ear.

UNEXPECTED: See table on p. 85.

Weber test.

- *Rinne test*
  Place base of vibrating tuning fork against mastoid bone, note seconds until sound is no longer heard; then quickly move fork 1 to 2 cm (½-1 inch) from auditory canal and note seconds until sound is no longer heard. Repeat with other ear.

EXPECTED: Measurement of air-conducted sound twice as long as measurement of bone-conducted sound.

UNEXPECTED: See table on p. 85.

Rinne test. **A,** Tuning fork against mastoid bone. **B,** Tuning fork near ear.

TECHNIQUE   FINDINGS

Interpretation of Tuning Fork Tests

	WEBER TEST	RINNE TEST
Expected findings	No lateralization, but will lateralize to ear occluded by patient	Air conduction heard longer than bone conduction by 2:1 ratio (Rinne positive)
Conductive hearing loss	Lateralization to deaf ear unless sensorineural loss	Bone conduction heard longer than air conduction in affected ear (Rinne negative)
Sensorineural hearing loss	Lateralization to better hearing ear unless conductive loss	Air conduction heard longer than bone conduction in affected ear, but <2:1 ratio

Nose and Sinuses

Inspect external nose

- *Shape/size*

EXPECTED: Smooth. Columella directly midline, width is not greater than diameter of a naris.
UNEXPECTED: Swelling or depression of nasal bridge. Transverse crease at junction of nose cartilage and bone.

- *Color*

EXPECTED: Conforms to face color.

- *Nares*

EXPECTED: Oval. Symmetrically positioned.
UNEXPECTED: Asymmetry, narrowing, discharge, nasal flaring on inspiration.

Palpate ridge and soft tissues of nose

Place one finger on each side of nasal arch and gently palpate from nasal bridge to tip.

EXPECTED: Firm and stable structures.
UNEXPECTED: Displacement of bone and cartilage, tenderness, or masses.

TECHNIQUE	FINDINGS
Evaluate patency of nares	
Occlude one naris with finger on side of nose and ask patient to breathe through nose. Repeat with other naris.	EXPECTED: Noiseless, easy breathing. UNEXPECTED: Noisy breathing; occlusion.

Inspect nasal mucosa and nasal septum

Carefully tilt back the patient's head and gently insert speculum without overdilating naris or touching nasal septum.

- *Color*

EXPECTED: Mucosa and turbinates deep pink and glistening.
UNEXPECTED: Increased redness of mucosa or localized redness and swelling in vestibule. Turbinates bluish gray or pale pink.

- *Shape*

EXPECTED: Septum close to midline and fairly straight, thicker anteriorly than posteriorly. Inferior and middle turbinates visible.
UNEXPECTED: Asymmetry of posterior nasal cavities, septal deviation.

- *Condition*

EXPECTED: Possibly film of clear discharge on septum. Possibly hairs in vestibule. Turbinates firm consistency.
UNEXPECTED: Discharge, bleeding, crusting, masses, or lesions. Swollen, boggy turbinates. Perforated septum. Polyps.

Sense of Smell

See Chapter 20.

TECHNIQUE   FINDINGS

Inspect frontal and maxillary sinus area

UNEXPECTED: Swelling on face over sinus areas.

Frontal sinuses
Ethmoid sinuses
Sphenoid sinus
Maxillary sinuses

Sinuses.

Palpate frontal and maxillary sinuses

Press thumbs up under bony brow on each side of nose. Palpate with thumbs or index and middle fingers just below the cheekbones.

EXPECTED: Nontender on palpation.
UNEXPECTED: Tenderness or pain, swelling.

Mouth

Inspect and palpate lips with mouth closed

Have patient remove lipstick (if applicable).

- *Symmetry*

EXPECTED: Symmetric vertically and horizontally at rest and while moving.
UNEXPECTED: Asymmetric.

- *Color*

EXPECTED: Pink in persons with lighter skin, more bluish in persons with darker skin, distinct border between lips and facial skin.
UNEXPECTED: Pallor, circumoral pallor, bluish purple, or cherry red.

TECHNIQUE	FINDINGS
• *Condition*	EXPECTED: Smooth. UNEXPECTED: Dry, cracked; deep fissures in mouth corners, swelling; lesions; plaques; vesicles; nodules, ulcerations; or round, oval, or irregular bluish-gray macules.

Inspect teeth

• *Occlusion*
Have patient clench teeth
and smile with lips spread.

EXPECTED: Upper molars fit
into the groove on lower molars. Premolars and canines
interlock fully. Upper incisors
slightly override lower
incisors.
UNEXPECTED: Malocclusion.
Protrusion of upper incisors
(overbite). Protrusion of lower
incisors. Problems with bite.

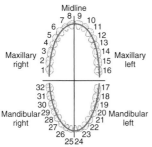

*Teeth occlusion line and individual tooth
numbers. (From Miyasaki-Ching, 1997.)*

• *Color*

EXPECTED: Ivory, stained
yellow or brown.
UNEXPECTED: Discolorations
on crown may indicate caries.

• *Condition*

EXPECTED: 32 teeth, firmly
anchored.
UNEXPECTED: Caries and loose
or missing teeth.

Inspect buccal mucosa

Have patient remove any dental
appliances and then partially
open mouth. Use tongue blade
and bright light to assess.

TECHNIQUE	FINDINGS
• *Color*	EXPECTED: Pinkish red, patchy pigmented mucosa in individuals with dark skin. UNEXPECTED: Deeply pigmented. Whitish or pinkish scars.
• *Condition*	EXPECTED: Smooth and moist. Whitish yellow or whitish pink Stensen duct. Fordyce spots (yellow-white raised lesions). UNEXPECTED: Adherent thickened white patch; white, round, or oval ulcerative lesions; red spot at opening of Stensen duct; stones or exudate from Stensen duct.

Inspect and palpate gingiva

Use gloves to palpate.

• *Color*	EXPECTED: Slightly stippled and pink, may be more hyperpigmented in individuals with dark skin.
• *Condition*	EXPECTED: Clearly defined, tight margin at each tooth. Gingival enlargement with pregnancy, puberty, certain medications. UNEXPECTED: Inflammation, swelling, bleeding, or lesions under dentures or on gingiva; induration, thickening, masses, or tenderness. Enlarged crevices between teeth and gum margins. Pockets containing debris at tooth margins.

Inspect tongue

• *Size/symmetry* Ask patient to extend tongue.	EXPECTED: Midline, no fasciculations. UNEXPECTED: Atrophied, deviation to one side.
• *Color*	EXPECTED: Dull red.

TECHNIQUE	FINDINGS
• *Dorsum surface* Have patient extend tongue and hold extended.	EXPECTED: Moist and glistening. Anterior: smooth yet roughened surface with papillae and small fissures. Posterior: smooth, slightly uneven or rugated surface with thinner mucosa than anterior. Possibly geographic. UNEXPECTED: Smooth, red, slick; hairy; swollen; coated; ulcerated; fasciculations; or limitation of movement.
• *Ventral surface and floor of mouth* Have patient touch tip of tongue to palate behind upper incisors.	EXPECTED: Ventral surface pink and smooth with large veins between frenulum and fimbriated folds. Wharton ducts apparent on each side of frenulum. UNEXPECTED: Difficulty touching hard palate. Swelling, varicosities, ranula (mucocele).
• *Lateral borders* Wrap tongue with gauze and pull to each side. Scrape white or red margins to remove food particles.	UNEXPECTED: Leukoplakia or any other fixed lesion, ulceration.

Inspecting lateral border of tongue.

Palpate tongue and floor of mouth

EXPECTED: Smooth and even texture.
UNEXPECTED: Lumps, nodules, induration, ulcerations, or thickened white patches.

TECHNIQUE	FINDINGS

Inspect palate and uvula

Have patient tilt head back.

- *Color and landmarks*

EXPECTED: Hard palate (whitish and dome-shaped with transverse rugae) contiguous with pinker soft palate. Uvula at midline. Bony protuberance of hard palate at midline (torus palatinus).
UNEXPECTED: Nodule on palate, not at midline.

- *Movement*
  Ask patient to say "ah" while observing soft palate.
  Depress tongue if necessary.

EXPECTED: Soft palate rises symmetrically, with uvula remaining in midline.
UNEXPECTED: Failure of soft palate to rise bilaterally. Uvula deviation. Bifid uvula.

Inspect oropharynx

Depress tongue with tongue blade.

- *Tonsils*
  Inspect the tonsillar pillars and size of tonsils.

EXPECTED: Tonsils, if present, blend into pink color of pharynx. Possible crypts in tonsils where cellular debris and food particles collect.
UNEXPECTED: Tonsils projecting beyond limits of tonsillar pillars. Tonsils red, enlarged, covered with exudate.

- *Posterior wall of pharynx*

EXPECTED: Smooth, glistening, pink mucosa with some small, irregular spots of lymphatic tissue and small blood vessels.
UNEXPECTED: Red bulge adjacent to tonsil extending beyond midline. Yellowish mucoid film in pharynx.

TECHNIQUE	FINDINGS
Elicit gag reflex	
Prepare patient and touch posterior wall of pharynx on each side.	EXPECTED: Bilateral response. UNEXPECTED: Unequal response or no response.

AIDS TO DIFFERENTIAL DIAGNOSIS

Differentiating Between Otitis Externa, Acute Otitis Media, and Middle-Ear Effusion

SIGNS AND SYMPTOMS	OTITIS EXTERNA	ACUTE OTITIS MEDIA	OTITIS MEDIA WITH EFFUSION
Initial symptoms	Itching in ear canal	Abrupt onset, fever, irritability, feeling of blockage	Sticking or cracking sound on yawning or swallowing; no signs of acute infection
Pain	Intense with movement of pinna or chewing	Deep-seated earache that interferes with activity or sleep, pulling at ear	Discomfort; feeling of fullness
Discharge	Watery, then purulent and thick, mixed with pus and epithelial cells; musty, foul smelling	Only if tympanic membrane ruptures or through tympanostomy; tube; foul smelling	Uncommon
Hearing	Conductive loss caused by exudate and swelling of ear canal	Conductive loss as middle ear fills with pus	Conductive loss as middle ear fills with fluid
Inspection	Canal is red, edematous; tympanic membrane is obscured	Tympanic membrane with distinct erythema, thickened or clouding, bulging; limited movement to positive and negative pressure, air–fluid level, and/or bubbles	Tympanic membrane is retracted or bulging, yellowish; impaired mobility; air–fluid level and/or bubbles

SUBJECTIVE DATA	OBJECTIVE DATA
Otitis Externa	
Swimming underwater, water retained in ear canal.	See differential diagnosis table on p. 92.
Otitis Media With Effusion	
Upper respiratory infection, ear feels full, reduced hearing.	See differential diagnosis table on p. 92.
Acute Otitis Media	
Recent upper respiratory infection, fever, ear pain or pressure, reduced hearing.	See differential diagnosis table on p. 92.
Sinusitis	
Upper respiratory infection worsens or persists after 7 to 10 days, headache, facial pain or pressure, tooth pain, nasal discharge or congestion, persistent cough (worse at night).	Fever, tenderness of sinuses, swelling over orbit or sinus; purulent nasal discharge; dull or opaque transillumination; may also have no physical findings.
Acute Bacterial Pharyngitis	
Sore throat, referred pain to ears, dysphagia, fever, fetid breath, malaise, abdominal pain, rash.	Tonsils are red and swollen; crypts filled with purulent exudate; enlarged anterior cervical lymph nodes; palatal petechiae.
Peritonsillar Abscess	
Difficulty and painful swallowing, severe sore throat with pain radiating to ear, fever, malaise.	Drooling, unilateral red and swollen tonsil and adjacent soft palate; tonsil, may appear pushed forward or backward, possibly displacing uvula; muffled voice, fetid breath, trismus, enlarged cervical lymph nodes.
Retropharyngeal Abscess	
Recent upper respiratory infection, pain in neck and jaw referred to ear, anxious, limited neck movement, drooling, poor appetite.	Fever, restlessness, pain with lateral neck movement, lateral pharyngeal wall is distorted medially, trismus, respiratory distress, muffled voice.

SUBJECTIVE DATA	OBJECTIVE DATA

Oral Cancer

Uses tobacco products, painless sore in mouth that does not heal; often discovered by health care provider or dentist.

Ulcerative lesion (red or white) on lateral border of tongue, floor of mouth, or other mucosa. Firm nonmobile mass, tooth mobility when no periodontal disease present; cervical lymphadenopathy.

Periodontal Disease

Red, swollen gums that easily bleed, tender gums, loose teeth, teeth sensitive to temperature.

Plaque and tartar buildup on teeth, deep pockets between teeth and gum margins, loose or missing teeth, halitosis.

PEDIATRIC VARIATIONS

EXAMINATION

Place infant in supine or prone position so head can be turned side to side. Position young child on caregiver's lap.

TECHNIQUE	FINDINGS

Ears

Inspect tympanic membrane

In infants, pull auricle downward and back to straighten canal.

EXPECTED: Tympanic membrane may be mildly red from crying. Other signs of infection should not be seen (bulging, limited mobility).

Assess hearing

To conduct an informal assessment, use a bell, whisper, or rub your fingers together to create a sound stimulus.

EXPECTED: For infants, see table on p. 95. Young children should turn toward sound consistently. When asked, children should repeat words whispered.

Sequences of Expected Hearing and Speech Response in Infants

AGE	RESPONSE
Birth to 3 mo	Startles, wakes, or cries when hearing a loud sound; quiets to parent's voice; makes vowel sounds "oh" and "ah."
4 to 6 mo	Turns head toward interesting sound; moves eyes in direction of sound but may not always recognize location of sound; responds to parent's voice; enjoys sound-producing toys; starts babbling and cooing.
7 to 12 mo	Responds to own name, telephone ringing, and person's voice, even if not loud; localizes sounds on all planes by turning eyes and head toward sound; babbles with short and long strings of sounds; begins to imitate speech sounds.

Modified from American Speech Language and Hearing Association: *How Does Your Child Hear and Talk?*, 2012. Retrieved from http://www.asha.org/public/speech/development/01.htm.

TECHNIQUE	FINDINGS

Nose and Sinuses

Evaluate patency of nares

With infant's mouth closed or with infant sucking on bottle or pacifier, occlude one naris and then the other. Observe respiratory pattern.

EXPECTED: Breathes easily; obligatory nose breathing until 2 to 3 mo of age.

Ethmoid sinuses

Sphenoid sinus

Maxillary sinus

Pediatric sinuses.

TECHNIQUE	FINDINGS

Mouth

Inspect and palpate lips with mouth closed

| | EXPECTED: Drooling in infants age 6 wk to 6 mo, sucking calluses in newborns.
UNEXPECTED: Drooling persistent after age 6 mo not associated with teething or drooling beyond 2 years of age. |

Inspect teeth

| Ask child to let you see his or her teeth. | EXPECTED: 0 to 20 teeth until age 6 years. Permanent teeth start erupting around age 6 years.
UNEXPECTED: Natal teeth. |

Inspect buccal mucosa

| | EXPECTED: In infants, nonadherent white patches (milk).
UNEXPECTED: In infants, adherent white patches. |

Inspect and palpate gingiva

| | EXPECTED: In infants up to 2 mo, pearl-like retention cysts. |

Inspect and palpate hard palate

| | EXPECTED: Strong suck and Epstein pearls in young infants.
UNEXPECTED: No cleft of hard or soft palate. |

AIDS TO DIFFERENTIAL DIAGNOSIS

SUBJECTIVE DATA	OBJECTIVE DATA

Cleft Lip and Palate

| Difficulty sucking, formula comes out of nose, failure to gain weight. | Unilateral or bilateral fissure or cleft in lip, hard palate, or soft palate that extends into the nasal cavity. |

Sample Documentation

Subjective. A 55-year-old man has concerns about hearing loss for the past few months; it is particularly difficult to hear people talking. He has difficulty hearing on the phone and when in conversations with multiple people talking. He hears "noise" in both ears when trying to go to sleep at night. There is no ear pain or discharge, no nasal discharge or sinus pain, no mouth lesions or masses, no recent dental problems, no sore throat, and no head trauma or exposure to ototoxic medications.

Objective

Ears: Auricles in alignment without masses, lesions, or tenderness. Canals totally obstructed by cerumen bilaterally. After irrigation, tympanic membranes are pearly gray, noninjected, intact, with bony landmarks and light reflex visualized bilaterally. No evidence of fluid or retraction. Conversational hearing appropriate. Able to hear whispered voice. Weber—lateralizes equally to both ears; Rinne—air conduction greater than bone conduction bilaterally (30 sec/15 sec).

Nose: No discharge or polyps, mucosa pink and moist, septum midline, patent bilaterally. No edema over frontal or maxillary sinuses. No sinus tenderness to palpation.

Mouth: Buccal mucosa pink and moist without lesions. Twenty-six teeth present in various states of repair. Lower second molars (18, 30) absent bilaterally. Gingiva pink and firm. Tongue midline with no tremors or fasciculation.

Pharynx: Clear without erythema; tonsils 1+ without exudate. Uvula rises evenly and gag reflex is intact. No hoarseness.

10 Chest and Lungs

Equipment

- Drape
- Skin-marking pencil
- Ruler and tape measure
- Stethoscope with bell and diaphragm

EXAMINATION

Have patient sit, disrobed to waist.

TECHNIQUE	FINDINGS

Chest and Lungs

Inspect front and back of chest

See thoracic landmarks.

- *Size/shape/symmetry*
- *Landmarks*

  EXPECTED: Supernumerary nipples possible (can be clue to other congenital abnormalities, particularly in white individuals).

- *Compare anteroposterior diameter with transverse diameter*

  EXPECTED: Ribs prominent, clavicles prominent superiorly, sternum usually flat and free of abundance of overlying tissue. Chest somewhat asymmetric. Anteroposterior diameter often half of transverse diameter.
  UNEXPECTED: Barrel chest, posterior or lateral deviation, pigeon chest, or funnel chest.

- *Assess nails, lips, nares*

  UNEXPECTED: Clubbed fingernails (usually symmetric and painless; may indicate disease, may be hereditary), pursed lips, flared alae nasi.

TECHNIQUE	FINDINGS
• *Color* Assess skin, lips, and nails.	UNEXPECTED: Superficial venous patterns. Cyanosis or pallor of lips or nails.
• *Breath*	UNEXPECTED: Malodorous.

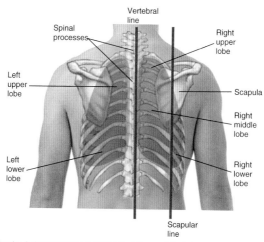

Thoracic landmarks. **A,** *Anterior thorax.* **B,** *Right lateral thorax.* **C,** *Posterior thorax.*

TECHNIQUE	FINDINGS

Evaluate respirations

- *Rhythm or pattern and rate*
  See patterns of respiration in the following figure.

EXPECTED: Breathing easy, regular, without distress. Pattern even. Rate 12-16 respirations/min. Ratio of respirations to heartbeats about 1:4.
UNEXPECTED: Dyspnea, orthopnea, paroxysmal nocturnal dyspnea, platypnea, tachypnea, hypopnea. Use of accessory muscles, retractions.

Normal	Regular and comfortable at a rate of 12-20 per minute	Air trapping	Increasing difficulty in getting breath out
Bradypnea	Slower than 12 breaths per minute	Cheyne-Stokes	Varying periods of increasing depth interspersed with apnea
Tachypnea	Faster than 20 breaths per minute	Kussmaul	Rapid, deep, labored
Hyperventilation (hyperpnea)	Faster than 20 breaths per minute, deep breathing	Biot	Irregularly interspersed periods of apnea in a disorganized sequence of breaths
Sighing	Frequently interspersed deeper breath	Ataxic	Significant disorganization with irregular and varying depths of respiration

Patterns of respiration. The horizontal axis indicates the relative rates of these patterns. The vertical swings of the lines indicate the relative depth of respiration.

- *Inspiration/expiration ratio*

UNEXPECTED: Air trapping, prolonged expiration.

Inspect chest movement with breathing

- *Symmetry*

EXPECTED: Chest expansion bilaterally symmetric.
UNEXPECTED: Asymmetry. Unilateral or bilateral bulging. Bulging on expiration.

TECHNIQUE	FINDINGS

Listen to respiration sounds audible without stethoscope

EXPECTED: Generally broncho-vesicular.
UNEXPECTED: Crepitus, stridor, wheezes.

Palpate thoracic muscles and skeleton

- *Symmetry/condition*

EXPECTED: Bilateral symmetry. Some elasticity of rib cage, but sternum and xiphoid relatively inflexible and thoracic spine rigid.
UNEXPECTED: Pulsations, tenderness, bulges, depressions, unusual movement, unusual positions.

- *Thoracic expansion*
Stand behind patient. Place palms in light contact with posterolateral surfaces and thumbs along spinal processes at tenth rib, as shown in figure at right. Watch thumb divergence during quiet and deep breathing. Face patient; place thumbs along costal margin and xiphoid process with palms touching anterolateral chest. Watch thumb divergence during quiet and deep breathing.

EXPECTED: Symmetric expansion.
UNEXPECTED: Asymmetric expansion.

Palpating thoracic expansion. The thumbs are at the level of the tenth rib.

TECHNIQUE	FINDINGS
• *Sensations*	EXPECTED: Nontender sensations. UNEXPECTED: Crepitus or grating vibration.
• *Tactile fremitus* Ask patient to recite numbers or words while systematically palpating chest with palmar surfaces of fingers or ulnar aspect of clenched fist, using firm, light touch. Assess each area, front to back, side to side, lung apices. Compare sides.	EXPECTED: Great variability; generally, fremitus is more intense with males (lower-pitched voice). UNEXPECTED: Decreased or absent fremitus; increased fremitus (coarser, rougher); or gentle, more tremulous fremitus. Variation between similar positions on right and left thorax.

Note position of trachea

Using index finger or thumbs, palpate gently from suprasternal notch along upper edges of each clavicle and in spaces above, to inner borders of sternocleidomastoid muscles.	EXPECTED: Spaces equal side to side. Trachea midline directly above suprasternal notch. Possible slight deviation to right. UNEXPECTED: Significant deviation or tug. Pulsations.

Perform percussion on chest

Percuss as shown in the following figure. Compare all areas bilaterally, following a sequence such as shown in figures on p. 103.
See table on p. 103 for common tones, intensity, pitch, duration, and quality.

Method for percussion.

TECHNIQUE   FINDINGS

*Suggested sequence for systematic percussion and auscultation of the thorax. **A,** Posterior thorax. **B,** Right lateral thorax. **C,** Left lateral thorax. **D,** Anterior thorax. The pleximeter finger or the stethoscope is moved in the numeric sequence suggested; however, other sequences are possible.*

Percussion Tones Heard Over the Chest

TYPE OF TONE	INTENSITY	PITCH	DURATION	QUALITY
Resonant	Loud	Low	Long	Hollow
Flat	Soft	High	Short	Extremely dull
Dull	Medium	Medium-high	Medium	Thudlike
Tympanic	Loud	High	Medium	Drumlike
Hyperresonant*	Very loud	Very low	Longer	Booming

*Hyperresonance is unexpected in adults. It represents air trapping, which occurs in obstructive lung diseases.

TECHNIQUE	FINDINGS
• *Thorax* Have patient sit with head bent and arms folded in front while percussing posterior thorax, then with arms raised overhead while percussing lateral and anterior chest. Percuss at 4- to 5-cm intervals over intercostal spaces, moving superior to inferior, medial to lateral. The female breast may obscure findings. You or patient may need to shift the breast, but pay careful attention to modesty.	EXPECTED: Resonance over all areas of lungs, dull over heart and liver, spleen, areas of thorax. UNEXPECTED: Hyperresonance, dullness, or flatness.
• *Diaphragmatic excursion* Ask patient to breathe deeply and hold breath. Percuss along scapular line on one side until tone changes from resonant to dull. Mark skin. Allow patient to breathe normally, then repeat on other side. Have patient take several breaths, then exhale as much as possible and hold. On each side, percuss up from mark to change from dull to resonant. Tell patient to resume breathing comfortably. Measure excursion distance.	EXPECTED: 3 to 5 cm (higher on right than left). UNEXPECTED: Limited descent.

Measuring diaphragmatic excursion. Excursion distance is usually 3 to 5 cm.

TECHNIQUE	FINDINGS

Auscultate chest with stethoscope diaphragm, apex to base

- *Intensity, pitch, duration, and quality of breath sounds* Have patient breathe slowly and deeply through mouth. Follow set auscultation sequence, holding stethoscope as shown in the following figure.
- Ask patient to sit upright:
  - (1) with head bent and arms folded in front while auscultating posterior thorax.
  - (2) with arms raised overhead while auscultating lateral chest.
  - (3) with arms down and shoulders back while auscultating anterior chest.

  Listen during inspiration and expiration. Auscultate downward from apex to base at intervals of several centimeters, making side-to-side comparisons.

EXPECTED: See expected breath sounds in table on p. 106. UNEXPECTED: Amphoric or cavernous breathing. Sounds difficult to hear or absent. Crackles, rhonchi, wheezes, or pleural friction rub, as described in box on pp. 106-107.

Auscultation with a stethoscope.

TECHNIQUE	FINDINGS
• *Vocal resonance* Ask patient to recite numbers or words.	EXPECTED: Muffled and indistinct sounds. UNEXPECTED: Bronchophony, whispered pectoriloquy, or egophony.

Characteristics of Expected Breath Sounds

SOUND	CHARACTERISTICS	FINDINGS
Vesicular	Heard over most of lung fields; low pitch; soft and short expirations; will be accentuated in a thin person or a child and diminished in overweight or very muscular patient.	
Bronchovesicular	Heard over main bronchus area and over upper right posterior lung field; medium pitch; expiration equals inspiration.	
Bronchotracheal (tubular)	Heard only over trachea; high pitch; loud and long expirations, often somewhat longer than inspiration.	

Adventitious Breath Sounds

Fine crackles: High-pitched, discrete, discontinuous crackling sounds heard during end of inspiration; not cleared by cough.

Medium crackles: Lower, more moist sound heard during midstage of inspiration; not cleared by cough.

Coarse crackles: Loud, bubbly noise heard during inspiration; not cleared by cough.

Rhonchi (sonorous wheeze): Loud, low, coarse sounds, like a snore, most often heard continuously during inspiration or expiration; coughing may clear sound (usually means mucus accumulation in trachea or large bronchi).

Wheeze (sibilant wheeze): Musical noise sounding like a squeak; most often heard continuously during inspiration or expiration; usually louder during expiration.

Pleural friction rub: Dry rubbing or grating sound, usually caused by inflammation of pleural surfaces; heard during inspiration or expiration; loudest over lower lateral anterior surface.

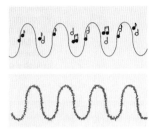

AIDS TO DIFFERENTIAL DIAGNOSIS

SUBJECTIVE DATA	OBJECTIVE DATA

Pleural Effusion

Cough with progressive dyspnea is the typical presenting concern. Pleuritic chest pain occurs with an inflammatory effusion.

Findings on auscultation and percussion vary with the amount of fluid present and with the position of the patient. These include dullness to percussion and tactile fremitus, which are the most useful findings for pleural effusion. When the fluid is mobile, it will gravitate to the most dependent position. In the affected areas, the breath sounds are muted and the percussion note is often hyperresonant in the area above the perfusion.

SUBJECTIVE DATA	OBJECTIVE DATA

Lung Cancer

Cough, wheezing, a variety of patterns of emphysema and atelectasis, pneumonitis, and hemoptysis. Peripheral tumors without airway obstruction may be asymptomatic.

Findings are based on the extent of the tumor and the patterns of its invasion and metastasis. With airway obstruction a postobstructive pneumonia can develop with consolidation. A malignant pleural effusion may develop with corresponding findings.

Pneumonia

Rapid onset (hours to days) of cough, pleuritic chest pain, and dyspnea. Sputum production is common with bacterial infection (see table on p. 109). Chills, fever, rigors, and nonspecific abdominal symptoms of nausea and vomiting may be present. Involvement of the right lower lobe can stimulate the tenth and eleventh thoracic nerves to cause right lower quadrant pain and simulate an abdominal process.

Febrile, tachypneic, and tachycardic. Crackles and rhonchi are common with diminished breath sounds. Egophony, bronchophony, and whispered pectoriloquy. Dullness to percussion occurs over the area of consolidation.

Asthma

Episodes of paroxysmal dyspnea and cough. Chest pain is common and, with it, a feeling of tightness. Episodes may last for minutes, hours, or days. May be asymptomatic between episodes.

Tachypnea with wheezing on expiration and inspiration. Expiration becomes more prolonged with labored breathing, fatigue, and anxious expression as airway resistance increases. Hypoxemia by pulse oximetry.

SUBJECTIVE DATA	OBJECTIVE DATA
Chronic Bronchitis	
Dyspnea may be present, although not severe. Cough and sputum production are impressive.	Wheezing and crackles. Hyperinflation with decreased breath sounds and a flattened diaphragm. Severe chronic bronchitis may result in right ventricular failure with dependent edema.
Emphysema	
Dyspnea is common even at rest. Cough is infrequent without much production of sputum.	Chest may be barrel shaped, and scattered crackles or wheezes may be heard. Overinflated lungs are hyperresonant on percussion. Inspiration is limited with a prolonged expiratory effort (i.e., >4 or 5 sec) to expel air.

Assessing Sputum

CAUSE	POSSIBLE SPUTUM CHARACTERISTICS
Bacterial infection	Yellow, green, rust colored (blood mixed with yellow sputum), clear, or transparent; purulent; blood streaked; mucoid, viscid
Viral infection	Mucoid, viscid; blood streaked (not common)
Chronic infectious disease	All of the above; particularly abundant in early morning; slight, intermittent blood streaking; occasionally large amounts of blood
Carcinoma	Slight, persistent blood streaking
Infarction	Blood clotted; large amounts of blood
Tuberculous cavity	Large amounts of blood

PEDIATRIC VARIATIONS

EXAMINATION

TECHNIQUE	FINDINGS

Chest and Lungs

Inspect front and back of chest

- *Compare anteroposterior diameter with transverse diameter*

EXPECTED: Infant's chest is expected to measure 2-3 cm less than head circumference.

Evaluate respirations

- *Rhythm or pattern and rate*

EXPECTED:

Age	Respirations/Min
Newborn	30 to 80
1 yr	20 to 40
3 yr	20 to 30
6 yr	16 to 22
10 yr	16 to 20
17 yr	12 to 16

Perform direct or indirect percussion on chest

- *Thorax*

EXPECTED: Hyperresonance may be heard in children.

Auscultate chest with stethoscope diaphragm, apex to base

- *Intensity, pitch, duration, and quality of breath sounds*

EXPECTED: In infants and children, expect transmitted breath sounds throughout chest. Vesicular sound is accentuated in a child. Absent or diminished breath sounds are harder to detect.

Sample Documentation

Subjective. A 45-year-old woman presents with cough and fever for 4 days. Cough is nonproductive, persistent, and worse when she lies down. She feels ill and short of breath. Her chest feels "heavy." Fever up to 38.3°C (101°F). Taking acetaminophen and nonprescription cough syrup without relief.

Objective. Pulse 104 beats per minute, temperature 38.2°C, blood pressure 122/82 mm Hg, respirations 32 breaths per minute and somewhat labored; no retractions or stridor. Minimal increase in anteroposterior diameter of chest, without kyphosis or other defect. Trachea in midline without tug. Thoracic expansion symmetric. No friction rubs or tenderness over ribs or other bony prominences. Over posterior left base, diminished tactile fremitus, dull percussion note, and on auscultation, crackles that do not clear with cough, diminished breath sounds. Remaining lung fields are clear and free of adventitious sounds, with resonant percussion tones. Diaphragmatic excursion 3 cm bilaterally.

Equipment

- Tangential light source
- Skin-marking pencil
- Stethoscope with bell and diaphragm
- Centimeter ruler

EXAMINATION

TECHNIQUE	FINDINGS

Heart

Inspect precordium

Have patient supine, and keep light source tangential.

- *Apical impulse*

EXPECTED: Visible about midclavicular line in fifth left intercostal space. Sometimes visible only with patient sitting.

UNEXPECTED: Visible in more than one intercostal space; exaggerated lifts or heaves.

Palpate precordium

- *Apical impulse*
  Have patient supine. With warm hands, gently feel precordium, using proximal halves of fingers held together or whole hand, as shown in figure on p. 113. Methodically move from apex to left sternal border, base, right sternal border, epigastrium, axillae.

EXPECTED: Gentle, brief impulse, palpable within radius of ≤1 cm, although often not felt.

UNEXPECTED: Heave or lift, loss of thrust, displacement to right or left; thrill.

TECHNIQUE	FINDINGS

Locate sensation in terms of its intercostal space and relationship to midsternal, midclavicular, axillary lines.

Percuss precordium (optional)

Begin by tapping at anterior axillary line, moving medially along intercostal spaces toward sternal borders until tone changes from resonance to dullness. Mark skin with marking pen.

EXPECTED: No change in tone before right sternal border; on left, loss of resonance generally close to point of maximal impulse at fifth intercostal space. Loss of resonance may outline left border of heart at second to fifth intercostal spaces.

Auscultate heart

Make certain patient is warm and relaxed. Isolate each sound and each pause in cycle, and then inch along with stethoscope. Systematically approach each of the five precordial areas, base to apex or apex to base, using each position shown in figures at right and below. Use diaphragm of stethoscope first, with firm pressure, then bell, with light pressure.

HEART

TECHNIQUE   FINDINGS

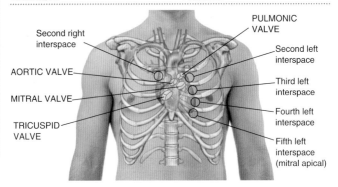

Second right interspace

PULMONIC VALVE

Second left interspace

AORTIC VALVE

Third left interspace

MITRAL VALVE

Fourth left interspace

TRICUSPID VALVE

Fifth left interspace (mitral apical)

- *Rate and rhythm*
  Assess overall rate and rhythm.

  EXPECTED: Rate 60 to 90 beats/min, regular rhythm.
  UNEXPECTED: Bradycardia, tachycardia, dysrhythmia.

- *S1*
  Ask patient to breathe comfortably, then hold breath in expiration.
     Listen for S1 (best heard toward apex) while palpating carotid pulse. Note intensity, variations, effect of respiration, splitting. Concentrate on systole, then diastole.

  EXPECTED: S1 usually heard as one sound and coincides with rise of carotid pulse. See table on p. 115.
  UNEXPECTED: Extra sounds or murmurs.

- *S2*
  Ask patient to breathe comfortably as you listen for S2 (best heard in aortic and pulmonic areas) to become two components during inspiration. Ask patient to inhale and hold breath.

  EXPECTED: S2 to become two components during inspiration. S2 to become an apparent single sound as breath is exhaled. See table on p. 115.

- *Splitting*

  EXPECTED: S2 splitting—greatest at peak of inspiration—varying from easily heard to nondetectable.

TECHNIQUE	FINDINGS
• *S3 and S4* If needed, ask patient to raise a leg to increase venous return or to grip your hand vigorously and repeatedly to increase venous return. • *Extra heart sounds*	EXPECTED: Both S3 and S4 quiet and difficult to hear. S3 has rhythm of Ken-tuc-ky; S4, Tenn-es-see. UNEXPECTED: Increased intensity (and ease of hearing) of either. UNEXPECTED: Extra heart sounds—snaps, clicks, friction rubs, murmurs. See the following table.

Assess characteristics of murmurs

Timing and duration, pitch, intensity, pattern, quality, location, radiation, respiratory phase variations.

Heart Sounds According to Auscultatory Area

	AORTIC	PULMONIC	SECOND PULMONIC	MITRAL	TRICUSPID
Pitch	S1 < S2	S1 < S2	S1 < S2	S1 > S2	S1 = S2
Loudness	S1 < S2	S1 < S2	S1 < S2*	S1 > S2†	S1 > S2
Duration	S1 < S2	S1 > S2	S1 < S2	S1 < S2	S1 = S2
S2 split	>Inhale	>Inhale	>Inhale	>Inhale‡	>Inhale
	<Exhale	<Exhale	<Exhale	<Exhale	<Exhale
A2	Loudest	Loud	Decreased		
P2	Decreased	Louder	Loudest		

*S1 is relatively louder in second pulmonic area than in aortic area.
†S1 may be louder in mitral area than in tricuspid area.
‡S2 split may not be audible in mitral area if P2 is inaudible.

Extra Heart Sounds

SOUND	DETECTION	DESCRIPTION
Increased S3	Bell at apex; patient left lateral recumbent	Early diastole, low pitch
Increased S4	Bell at apex; patient supine or semilateral	Late diastole or early systole, low pitch
Gallops	Bell at apex; patient supine or left lateral recumbent	Presystole, intense, easily heard

HEART

Extra Heart Sounds—cont'd

SOUND	DETECTION	DESCRIPTION
Mitral valve opening snap	Diaphragm medial to apex, may radiate to base; any position, second left intercostal	Early diastole briefly, before S3; high pitch, sharp snap or click; not affected by respiration; easily confused with S2
Ejection clicks	Diaphragm; patient sitting or supine	
Aortic valve	Diaphragm, right second intercostal space	Early systole, intense, high pitch; radiates, not affected by respirations
Pulmonary valve	Diaphragm; left second intercostal right space	Early systole, less intense than aortic click; intensifies on expiration, decreases on inspiration
Pericardial friction rub	Diaphragm, widely heard, sound clearest toward apex	May occupy all of systole and diastole; intense, grating, machinelike; may have three components and obliterate heart sounds; if only one or two components, may sound like murmur

AIDS TO DIFFERENTIAL DIAGNOSIS

SUBJECTIVE DATA	OBJECTIVE DATA
Left Ventricular Hypertrophy	
Initially asymptomatic, may cause shortness of breath or chest pain.	Vigorous, sustained lift palpable during ventricular systole, sometimes over broader area than usual (by ≥2 cm). Displacement of apical impulse can be well lateral of midclavicular line and downward.
Right Ventricular Hypertrophy	
Fatigue, shortness of breath, syncope may indicate more severe disease.	Lift along left sternal border in third and fourth left intercostal spaces accompanied by occasional systolic retraction at apex. Left ventricle displaced and turned posteriorly by enlarged right ventricle.

SUBJECTIVE DATA	OBJECTIVE DATA
Congestive Heart Failure	
May be left or right sided: Left sided is either systolic or diastolic. Fatigue, orthopnea, shortness of breath, edema.	Congestion in pulmonary or systemic circulation. Can develop gradually or suddenly with acute pulmonary or systemic edema.
Cor Pulmonale	
Tachypnea, fatigue, exertional dyspnea, cough hemoptysis.	Left parasternal systolic lift and loud S2 in pulmonic region, evidence of pulmonary disease.
Myocardial Infarction	
Deep substernal or visceral pain, often radiating to jaw, neck, left arm (although discomfort is sometimes mild); women may experience milder and different symptoms.	Dysrhythmias; S4 often present. Heart sounds distant, with soft, systolic, blowing murmur; pulse possibly thready; varied blood pressure (although hypertension usual in early phases).
Myocarditis	
Initially symptoms vague; fatigue, dyspnea, fever, palpitations. Symptoms may progress.	Cardiac enlargement, murmur, gallop rhythms, tachycardia, dysrhythmias, pulsus alternans.
Conduction Disturbances	
Transient weakness, syncope, strokelike episodes, palpitations.	Labile heart rates.
Atherosclerotic Heart Disease	
May be asymptomatic or cause angina pectoris, shortness of breath, and palpitations.	May cause myocardial insufficiency, dysrhythmias, congestive heart failure.

HEART

SUBJECTIVE DATA	OBJECTIVE DATA
Angina	
Substernal pain or intense pressure radiating at times to neck, jaws, arms, particularly left arm, often accompanied by shortness of breath, fatigue, diaphoresis, faintness, syncope. Cessation of activity may relieve pain.	No pathognomonic examination findings, tachycardia, hypertension, diaphoresis, decreased S1 intensity, S4.

Chest Pain

TYPE OF CHEST PAIN	CHARACTERISTICS
Anginal	Substernal; provoked by effort, emotion, eating; relieved by rest and/or nitroglycerin
Pleural	Precipitated by breathing or coughing; usually described as sharp
Esophageal	Burning, substernal, occasional radiation to shoulder; nocturnal occurrence, usually when lying flat; relief with food, antacids, sometimes nitroglycerin
From a peptic ulcer	Almost always infradiaphragmatic and epigastric; nocturnal occurrence and daytime attacks; should not be relieved by food; unrelated to activity
Biliary	Usually under right scapula, prolonged in duration; will trigger angina more often than mimic it
From arthritis/bursitis	Usually of hours' long duration; local tenderness and/or pain with movement
Cervical	Associated with injury; provoked by activity, persists after activity; painful on palpation and/or movement
Musculoskeletal (chest)	Intensified or provoked by movement, particularly twisting or costochondral bending; long lasting; often associated with local tenderness
Psychoneurotic	Associated with or occurring after anxiety; poorly described, located in intramammary region

PEDIATRIC VARIATIONS

EXAMINATION

TECHNIQUE	FINDINGS
Assess characteristics of murmurs	
Timing and duration, intensity, pattern, quality, location, radiation, respiratory phase variations.	In children it is necessary to distinguish innocent murmurs from organic murmurs caused by congenital defect or rheumatic fever.

AIDS TO DIFFERENTIAL DIAGNOSIS

SUBJECTIVE DATA	OBJECTIVE DATA

Chest Pain

Unlike in adults, chest pain in children and adolescents is seldom caused by a cardiac problem. It is very often difficult to find a cause, but trauma, exercise-induced asthma, and use of cocaine, even in a somewhat younger child, as in the adolescent and adult, should be among the considerations.

Examination is usually normal.

Congenital Defects

Tetralogy of Fallot

Dyspnea with feeding, poor growth, exercise intolerance, tetralogy spells.

Parasternal heave and precordial prominence, cyanosis, systolic ejection murmur heard over third intercostal space, sometimes radiating to left side of neck. Single S2.

Ventricular septal defect

Tachypnea, symptoms of right-sided congestive heart failure, poor growth, recurrent respiratory infections.

Arterial pulse small, jugular venous pulse unaffected, regurgitation occurs through septal defect, resulting in holosystolic murmur that is often loud, coarse, high pitched, best heard along left sternal border in third to fifth intercostal spaces. Distinct lift often discernible along left sternal border and apical area. Does not radiate to neck.

HEART

HEART

SUBJECTIVE DATA	OBJECTIVE DATA
Patent ductus arteriosus	
Asymptomatic if small; larger patent ductus arteriosi cause dyspnea on exertion.	Neck vessels dilate and pulsate, and pulse pressure wide. Harsh, loud, continuous murmur with machine-like quality, heard at first to third intercostal spaces and lower sternal border. Murmur usually unaltered by postural change.
Atrial septal defect	
Often asymptomatic, congestive heart failure in adults.	Systolic ejection murmur, best heard over pulmonic area that is diamond shaped, often loud, high in pitch, and harsh. May be accompanied by brief, rumbling, early diastolic murmur. Does not usually radiate beyond precordium. Systolic thrill may be felt over area of murmur along with palpable parasternal thrust. S2 may be split fairly widely. Particularly significant with palpable thrust and occasional radiation through to back.

Sample Documentation

Heart. No visible pulsations over precordium. Point of maximal impulse palpable at the fifth intercostals in the midclavicular line, 1 cm in diameter. No lifts, heaves, or thrills felt on palpation. S1 is crisp. Split S2 increases with inspiration. No audible S3, S4, murmur, click, or rub.

Blood Vessels

Equipment

- Tangential light source
- Stethoscope with bell and diaphragm
- Sphygmomanometer
- Centimeter ruler

EXAMINATION

TECHNIQUE   FINDINGS

Peripheral Arteries

Palpate arterial pulses in neck and extremities

Palpate carotid, brachial,
radial, femoral, popliteal,
dorsalis pedis, and posterior
tibial arteries, using distal
pads of second and third
fingers, as shown in following
figures and those on p. 123.

- *Characteristics*
  Compare characteristics
  bilaterally, as well as
  between upper and lower
  extremities.

EXPECTED: Femoral pulse as
strong as or stronger than radial
pulse.
UNEXPECTED: Femoral pulse
weaker than radial pulse or
absent. Alternating pulse (pulsus
alternans), pulsus bisferiens,
bigeminal pulse (pulsus bi-
geminus), bounding pulse, labile
pulse, paradoxical pulse (pulsus
paradoxus), pulsus differens,
tachycardia, trigeminal pulse
(pulsus trigeminus), or water-
hammer pulse (Corrigan pulse).

TECHNIQUE   FINDINGS

*Palpation of arterial pulses. **A**, Carotid. **B**, Brachial. **C**, Radial. **D**, Femoral. **E**, Popliteal.*
*F, Dorsalis pedis. **G**, Posterior tibial.*

- *Rate*

  EXPECTED: 60 to 90 beats/min.
  UNEXPECTED: Rate different from
  that observed during cardiac
  examination.

- *Rhythm*

  EXPECTED: Regular.
  UNEXPECTED: Irregular, either in
  a pattern or patternless.

- *Contour*

  EXPECTED: Smooth, rounded, or
  dome shaped.

BLOOD VESSELS

PULSE

Alternating pulse (pulsus alternans)

POSSIBLE CAUSE

Left ventricular failure
(More significant if
pulse slow)

A   Pulsus alternans is characterized by alternation of a pulsation of small amplitude with the
pulsation of large amplitude while the rhythm is regular.

Pulsus bisferiens

Aortic stenosis combined
with aortic insufficiency

B   Pulsus bisferiens is best detected by palpation of the carotid artery. This pulsation is
characterized by two main peaks. The first is termed percussion wave and the second, tidal
wave. Although the mechanism is not clear, the first peak is believed to be the pulse pressure
and the second, reverberation from the periphery.

Bigeminal pulse

Disorder of rhythm

C   Bigeminal pulsations result from a normal pulsation followed by a premature contraction. The
amplitude of the pulsation of the premature contraction is less than that of the normal pulsation.

Large, bounding pulse

Exercise
Anxiety
Fever
Hyperthyroidism
Aortic rigidity or
atherosclerosis

D   The large, bounding (also called hyperkinetic or strong) pulse is readily palpable. It does not
"fade out" and is not easily obliterated by the examining fingers. This pulse is recorded as 3+.

Paradoxic pulse (pulsus paradoxus)

Inspiration   Expiration   Inspiration

Premature cardiac contraction
Tracheobronchial obstruction
Bronchial asthma
Emphysema
Pericardial effusion
Constrictive pericarditis

E   Pulsus paradoxus is characterized by an exaggerated decrease (>10 mm Hg) in the amplitude of
pulsation during inspiration and increased amplitude during expiration. (See text for measurement
with sphygmomanometer.)

Water-hammer pulse (Corrigan pulse)

Patent ductus arteriosus
Aortic regurgitation

F   The water-hammer pulse (also known as collapsing) has a greater amplitude than expected, a
rapid rise to a narrow summit, and a sudden descent.

A-F, Pulse abnormalities.

- *Amplitude*

UNEXPECTED: Bounding, full,
diminished, or absent. Describe
on scale of 0 to 4:
0 = Absent, not palpable
1 = Diminished
2 = Expected
3 = Full, increased
4 = Bounding

TECHNIQUE	FINDINGS

Auscultate carotid and subclavian arteries; abdominal aorta; and renal, iliac, and femoral arteries for bruits

When auscultating the carotid vessels, you may at times need to ask patient to hold breath for a few heartbeats. Auscultate with bell of stethoscope.

UNEXPECTED: Transmitted murmurs, bruits.

Assess for arterial occlusion and insufficiency

- *Site*
  Assess for pain distal to possible occlusion.

UNEXPECTED: Dull ache accompanied by fatigue and often cramping; possible constant or excruciating pain. Weak, thready, or absent pulses; systolic bruits over arteries; loss of body warmth; localized pallor or cyanosis; delay in venous filling; or thin, atrophied skin, muscle atrophy, and loss of hair.

- *Degree of occlusion*
  Ask patient to lie supine. Elevate extremity, note degree of blanching, then ask patient to sit on edge of table or bed to lower extremity. Note time for maximal return of color when extremity is lowered.

EXPECTED: Slight pallor on elevation and return to full color as soon as leg becomes dependent.
UNEXPECTED: Delay of >2 sec.

Measure blood pressure

Measure in both arms at least once. Patient's arm should be slightly flexed and comfortably supported on table, pillow, or your hand.

EXPECTED: <120 mm Hg systolic and <80 mm Hg diastolic, with pulse pressure of 30 to 40 mm Hg (sometimes to 50 mm Hg). Reading between arms may vary by as much as 10 mm Hg. Prehypertension is now defined as a blood pressure between 120 and 139 mm Hg systolic or 80 and 89 mm Hg diastolic.
UNEXPECTED: Hypertension (see Chapter 2).

BLOOD VESSELS

Peripheral Veins

Assess jugular venous pressure

Ask patient to recline at 45-degree angle. With tangential light, observe the jugular vein. As shown in figure below, use a centimeter ruler to measure vertical distance between midaxillary line and highest level of jugular vein distention.

EXPECTED: Pressure ≤9 cm H_2O, bilaterally symmetric.
UNEXPECTED: Abnormal elevation, distention or distention on one side.

Assess for venous obstruction and insufficiency

Inspect extremities, with patient both standing and supine.

- *Affected area*

  UNEXPECTED: Constant pain with swelling and tenderness over muscles, engorgement of superficial veins, cyanosis.

- *Thrombosis*
  Examine the patient's calf for pain, swelling erythema.

  UNEXPECTED: Redness, thickening, tenderness along superficial vein. Calf swelling.

- *Edema*
  Press index finger over bony prominence of tibia or medial malleolus for several seconds.

  UNEXPECTED: Orthostatic (pitting) edema; thickening and ulceration of skin possible.

Grade edema from 1+ to 4+ as follows:

1+ = Slight pitting, no visible distortion, disappears rapidly
2+ = Deeper than 1+ and disappears in 10-15 sec
3+ = Noticeably deep and may last >1 min, with dependent extremity full and swollen
4+ = Very deep and lasts 2 to 5 min, with grossly distorted dependent extremity

BLOOD VESSELS

TECHNIQUE	FINDINGS
• *Varicose veins* If suspected, have patient stand on toes 10 times in succession.	EXPECTED: Pressure from toe standing disappears in seconds. UNEXPECTED: Veins dilated and swollen; often tortuous when extremities are dependent and pressure does not quickly disappear.
• *If varicose veins are present, assess venous incompetence with Trendelenburg test:* Ask patient to lie supine, lift leg above heart level until veins empty, then quickly lower leg.	UNEXPECTED: Rapid filling of veins.
• *Evaluate patency of deep veins with Perthes test:* Ask patient to lie supine. Elevate extremity, and occlude subcutaneous veins with tourniquet just above knee. Then ask patient to walk.	UNEXPECTED: Superficial veins fail to empty.
• *Evaluate direction of blood flow and presence of compensatory circulation:* Put affected limb in dependent position, then empty or strip vein. Release pressure of one finger nearest heart to assess blood flow; if necessary, repeat and release pressure of other finger.	UNEXPECTED: Stripped vessel fills before pressure is released by distal finger, or blood refills entire vein when pressure is released by proximal finger.

AIDS TO DIFFERENTIAL DIAGNOSIS

OBJECTIVE DATA	SUBJECTIVE DATA
Arterial Aneurysm	
Generally asymptomatic until they dissect or compress an adjacent structure. With dissection, the patient may describe a severe ripping pain.	Pulsatile swelling along the course of an artery. Occurs most commonly in the aorta, although renal, femoral, and popliteal arteries are also common sites. A thrill or bruit may be evident over the aneurysm.

OBJECTIVE DATA	SUBJECTIVE DATA
Venous Thrombosis	
Tenderness along the iliac vessels or the femoral canal, in the popliteal space, or over the deep calf veins. Deep vein thrombosis in the femoral and pelvic circulations may be asymptomatic. Pulmonary embolism may occur without warning.	Swelling may be distinguished only by measuring and comparing the circumference of the upper and lower legs bilaterally. There may be minimal ankle edema, low-grade fever, and tachycardia. Homan sign can be helpful but is not absolutely reliable in suggesting deep vein thrombosis.
Raynaud Phenomenon	
Involved areas will feel cold and achy, which improves on rewarming. In secondary Raynaud phenomenon, there can be intense pain and digital ischemia with necrosis at the tips.	With primary Raynaud phenomenon, there is triphasic demarcated skin pallor (white), cyanosis (blue), and reperfusion (red) within the extremities. The vasospasm may last from minutes to less than an hour. In secondary Raynaud phenomenon, ulcers may appear on the tips of the digits, and eventually the skin over the digits can appear smooth, shiny, and tight from loss of subcutaneous tissue.

PEDIATRIC VARIATIONS

EXAMINATION

TECHNIQUE	FINDINGS
Palpate Arterial Pulses in Distal Extremities (see Chapter 2)	
Auscultate arteries for bruits	
	EXPECTED: In children, it is not unusual to hear a venous hum over internal jugular veins. There is usually no pathologic significance.
Measure blood pressure (see Chapter 2)	

AIDS TO DIFFERENTIAL DIAGNOSIS

SUBJECTIVE DATA	OBJECTIVE DATA

Coarctation of the Aorta

Most patients are asymptomatic unless severe hypertension or vascular insufficiency develops. In those settings, patients may experience symptoms of heart failure or vascular insufficiency of an involved upper extremity with activity.

Differences in systolic blood pressure readings when the radial and femoral pulses are palpated simultaneously.

Sample Documentation

Vessels. Neck veins not distended. Both A and V waves are visualized. Jugular venous pressure (JVP) is 4 cm water at 45 degrees. Arterial pulses equal and symmetric, testing on a scale of 1 to 4.

	C	B	R	F	P	PT	DP
L	2+	2+	2+	2+	2+	2+	2+
R	2+	2+	2+	2+	2+	2+	2+

Vessels soft. No bruits are audible.

Extremities. No edema, skin, or nail changes. Superficial varicosities noted in both lower extremities. No areas of tenderness to palpation.

Breasts and Axillae

Equipment

- Ruler (if mass detected)
- Flashlight with transilluminator (if mass detected)
- Glass slide and cytologic fixative (if nipple discharge is present)
- Small pillow or folded towel

EXAMINATION

Describe any breast mass or lump that you encounter using the following characteristics:

- Location: clock positions and distance from nipple
- Size (in centimeters): length, width, thickness
- Shape: round, discoid, lobular, stellate, regular or irregular
- Consistency: firm, soft, hard
- Tenderness
- Mobility: movable (in what directions) or fixed to overlying skin or subadjacent fascia
- Borders: discrete or poorly defined
- Retraction: presence or absence of dimpling; altered contour

  All new solitary or dominant masses must be investigated with further diagnostic testing.

TECHNIQUE	FINDINGS

Patients With Female Breasts

With patient seated and arms hanging loosely, inspect both breasts

Inspect all quadrants and tail of Spence. If necessary, lift breasts with fingertips to expose lower and lateral aspects.

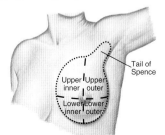

Tail of Spence

Upper inner | Upper outer

Lower inner | Lower outer

TECHNIQUE	FINDINGS
• *Size/shape/symmetry*	EXPECTED: Convex, pendulous, or conical. Long-standing asymmetry in size. UNEXPECTED: Asymmetry in position (nipples point in different directions); new asymmetry in size. Implants that have shifted. Surgical modification
• *Texture/contour*	EXPECTED: Smooth and uninterrupted. UNEXPECTED: Dimpling, retraction, or peau d'orange appearance. Changes or asymmetric appearance.
• *Skin color*	EXPECTED: Consistent color. UNEXPECTED: Areas of discoloration, erythema, or asymmetric appearance.
• *Venous patterns*	EXPECTED: Bilateral venous networks, although usually pronounced only in pregnant patients. UNEXPECTED: Unilateral network.
• *Markings*	EXPECTED: Long-standing nevi. Supernumerary nipples possible (but could be a clue to other congenital abnormalities). UNEXPECTED: Changing or tender nevi. Lesions.

Inspect areolae and nipples

• *Size/shape/symmetry*	EXPECTED: Areolae round or oval, bilaterally equal or nearly equal. Nipples bilaterally equal or nearly equal in size and usually everted, although one or both sometimes inverted. UNEXPECTED: Recent unilateral nipple inversion or retraction.

TECHNIQUE	FINDINGS
• *Color*	EXPECTED: Areolae and nipples pink to brown. UNEXPECTED: Nonhomogeneous in color.
• *Texture/contour*	EXPECTED: Areolae smooth, except for Montgomery tubercles. Nipples smooth or wrinkled. UNEXPECTED: Areolae with suppurative or tender Montgomery tubercles or with peau d'orange appearance. Nipples crusting, cracking, or with discharge.

With patient in the following positions, reinspect both breasts

• *Arms extended over head or flexed behind the neck*	EXPECTED: All positions breasts bilaterally symmetric with even contour.
• *Hands pressed on hips with shoulders rolled forward or pushed together in front*	UNEXPECTED: Dimpling, retraction, deviation, or fixation of breasts.
• *Seated and leaning over*	
• *Recumbent*	

With patient seated and arms hanging loosely, palpate breasts

Chest wall sweep. Place the palm of your right hand at the patient's right clavicle at the sternum. Sweep downward from the clavicle to the nipple, feeling for superficial lumps. Repeat the sweep until you have covered the entire right chest wall. Repeat the procedure using your left hand for the left chest wall.

EXPECTED: Tissue smooth, free of lumps.
UNEXPECTED: Lumps or nodules. Reassess with additional palpation and characterize any masses by location, size, shape, consistency, tenderness, mobility, delineation of borders, retraction. Use transillumination to assess presence of fluid in masses.

Bimanual digital palpation. Place one hand, palmar surface facing up, under the patient's right breast. Position your hand so that it acts as a flat surface against which to compress the breast tissue. Walk the fingers of the other hand across the breast tissue, feeling for lumps as you compress the tissue between your fingers and your flat hand. Repeat the procedure for the other breast.

EXPECTED: Tissue generally firm, nontender, free of lumps. During menstrual cycle, cyclic pattern of breast enlargement, increased nodularity, tenderness.
UNEXPECTED: Lumps or nodules. Reassess with additional palpation and characterize any masses by location, size, shape, consistency, tenderness, mobility, delineation of borders, retraction. Use transillumination to assess presence of fluid in masses.

BREASTS AND AXILLAE

TECHNIQUE	FINDINGS

With patient seated, palpate for lymph nodes

Axillary: Support patient's forearm with your contralateral arm and bring palm of examining hand flat into axilla. With palmar surface of fingers, reach deep into hollow, pushing firmly upward, then bring fingers down, rotating your fingers and gently rolling soft tissue against chest wall and axilla. Explore apex, medial, lateral aspects along rib cage; lateral aspects along upper surface of arm; and anterior and posterior walls of axilla. Repeat mirror image of this maneuver for the other axilla. *Supraclavicular area:* Hook fingers over clavicle and rotate over supraclavicular fossa while patient turns head toward same side and raises shoulder. *Infraclavicular area:* Palpate along the clavicle using a rotary motion with your fingers.

EXPECTED: Nodes not palpable. UNEXPECTED: Nodes, especially in supraclavicular area. Describe nodes by location, size, shape, consistency, tenderness, fixation, delineation of borders.

TECHNIQUE	FINDINGS

With patient supine, continue palpation of breast tissue

Have patient put one hand behind head. Place a towel under shoulder of same side. Compress breast tissue between fingers and chest wall, using rotary motion of fingers. Using finger pads, systematically palpate each breast in all four quadrants, including tail of Spence and over areolae. Push gently but firmly toward chest while rotating fingers clockwise or counterclockwise, following a vertical strip, concentric circle, or wedge pattern. At each point, press inward, using three depths of palpation: light, medium, and deep. Return to the nipple and with two fingers gently depress the tissue inward into the well behind the areola. Repeat palpation maneuvers for other breast.

EXPECTED: Tissue generally dense, firm, elastic but sometimes lobular. May be fine and granular in older women. Inframammary ridge may be felt along lower edge of breast. During menstrual cycle, cyclic pattern of breast enlargement, increased nodularity, tenderness. Implants may be present.
UNEXPECTED: Lumps or nodules, hardened tissue. Characterize any masses by location, size, shape, consistency, tenderness, mobility, delineation of borders, retraction. Use transillumination to assess presence of fluid in masses. Implants that have rupture or contracted.
EXPECTED: Fingers and tissue move easily inward.
UNEXPECTED: Lump, mass; absence of well behind areola.

TECHNIQUE	FINDINGS

Patients with Male Breasts
Inspect both breasts

- *Size/shape/symmetry*

EXPECTED: Even with chest wall. Sometimes convex (especially in overweight men).

- *Surface characteristics*

UNEXPECTED: Enlarged breasts.

Inspect areolae and nipples

- *Size/shape/symmetry*

EXPECTED: Areolae round or oval, bilaterally equal or nearly equal. Nipples bilaterally equal or nearly equal in size and usually everted, although one or both sometimes inverted.
UNEXPECTED: Recent unilateral nipple inversion or retraction.

- *Color*

EXPECTED: Areolae and nipples pink to brown.
UNEXPECTED: Nonhomogeneous in color.

- *Texture/contour*

EXPECTED: Areolae smooth, except for Montgomery tubercles. Nipples smooth or wrinkled.
UNEXPECTED: Areolae with suppurative or tender Montgomery tubercles or with peau d'orange appearance. Nipples crusting, cracking, or with discharge.

Palpate breasts and over areolae

- *Palpate briefly, following palpation steps for patients with female breasts*

EXPECTED: Thin layer of fatty tissue overlying muscle. Thick layer in obese men may give appearance of breast enlargement. Firm disk of glandular tissue sometimes evident.
UNEXPECTED: Lumps or nodules.

TECHNIQUE	FINDINGS

With patient seated and arms flexed at elbows, palpate for lymph nodes

- *Palpate as described for patients with female breasts.*

EXPECTED: Nodes not palpable.
UNEXPECTED: Nodes, especially in supraclavicular area. Describe nodes by location, size, shape, consistency, tenderness, fixation, delineation of borders.

AIDS TO DIFFERENTIAL DIAGNOSIS

SUBJECTIVE DATA	OBJECTIVE DATA

Fibrocystic Changes

Tender and painful breasts and/ or palpable lumps that fluctuate with menses; usually worse premenstrually.

Round, soft to firm, tense, mobile masses with well-delineated borders; usually tender; usually bilateral; multiple or single.

Fibroadenoma

Painless lumps that do not fluctuate with the menstrual cycle; may be asymptomatic with discovery on clinical breast examination or mammogram.

Round or discoid, firm, rubbery, mobile masses with well-delineated borders; usually nontender, usually bilateral, single; may be multiple; biopsy often performed to rule out carcinoma.

Malignant Breast Tumors

Painless lump, change in size, shape or contour of breast, axilla may be tender if lymph nodes involved; may be asymptomatic with discovery on clinical breast examination or mammogram.

Palpable mass that is usually single, unilateral, irregular, or stellate in shape; poorly delineated borders; fixed, hard, stonelike, and nontender; breast may have dimpling, retraction, prominent vasculature; skin may have peau d'orange or thickened appearance; nipple may be inverted or deviate in position.

SUBJECTIVE DATA	OBJECTIVE DATA
Intraductal Papillomas and Papillomatosis	
Spontaneous nipple discharge, usually unilateral; usually serous or bloody.	Single-duct unilateral nipple discharge provoked on physical examination.
Gynecomastia	
Breast enlargement in male individuals.	Smooth, firm, mobile, tender disk of breast tissue behind areola, unilaterally or bilaterally.
Mastitis	
Sudden onset of swelling, tenderness, redness, and heat in the breast; usually chills, fever.	Tender, hard breast mass, with an area of fluctuation, erythema, and heat; may have discharge of pus (suppuration).

PEDIATRIC VARIATIONS

EXAMINATION

TECHNIQUE	FINDINGS
Palpate and compress nipples	
	EXPECTED: Breast enlargement is not unusual in newborns. "Witch's milk" may be expressed.
Assess stage of pubertal development	
In female patients, assess the stage of breast development.	EXPECTED: The duration and tempo of each stage and sequence are quite variable between individuals. Tanner stages of breast development are shown on p. 10.

BREASTS AND AXILLAE

M₁—Tanner 1 (preadolescent). Only the nipple is raised above the level of the breast, as in the child.

M₂—Tanner 2. Budding stage; bud-shaped elevation of the areola; areola increased in diameter and surrounding area slightly elevated.

M₃—Tanner 3. Breast and areola enlarged. No contour separation.

M₄—Tanner 4. Increasing fat deposits. The areola forms a secondary elevation above that of the breast. This secondary mound occurs in approximately half of all girls and in some cases persists in adulthood.

M₅—Tanner 5 (adult stage). The areola is (usually) part of general breast contour and is strongly pigmented. Nipple projects.

Five stages of breast development in females. (Growth diagrams from Van Wieringen JC, Wafel-bakker F, Verbrugge HP, DeHaas JH: Netherlands: Second National Survey on 0-24-Year-Olds, Groningen, The Netherlands: Noordhoff Uitgevers BV, 1965.)

AIDS TO DIFFERENTIAL DIAGNOSIS

SUBJECTIVE DATA	OBJECTIVE DATA
Premature Thelarche	
Breast enlargement before onset of puberty.	Degree of enlargement varies from very slight to fully developed breasts. Usually bilateral. Other signs of sexual maturation may be absent.

Sample Documentation

Subjective. A 42-year-old woman noticed a "knot" in her right lower breast last week. Denies nipple discharge or skin changes. Reports normal mammogram last year. Has never had a breast lump before. Currently on last day of menses. Has breast tenderness just before menses but denies breast pain today. No family history of breast cancer.

Objective. Breasts moderate size, conical shape, left slightly larger than right. No skin lesions, contour smooth without dimpling or retraction; venous pattern symmetric. Nipples symmetric, without spontaneous discharge, depress into the wells easily. Montgomery tubercles bilaterally. Breasts diffusely nodular, particularly in upper outer quadrants. In right breast there is a 3- × 2-cm soft, mobile, nontender mass with discrete, well-defined borders at the 4-o'clock position 6 cm from the nipple. No supraclavicular, infraclavicular, or axillary lymphadenopathy.

14 Abdomen

Equipment

- Stethoscope
- Centimeter measuring tape
- Marking pen

EXAMINATION

Have patient in the supine position to start the examination. Approach the patient from the right side.

TECHNIQUE	FINDINGS
Inspect abdomen	
• *Skin color/characteristics*	EXPECTED: Usual color variations, such as paleness or tanning lines. Fine venous network (venous return toward head above umbilicus, toward feet below umbilicus). UNEXPECTED: Generalized color changes, such as jaundice or cyanosis. Glistening, taut appearance. Bluish periumbilical discoloration, bruises, other localized discoloration. Striae, lesions or nodules, a pearl-like enlarged umbilical node, scars.
• *Contour/symmetry* Begin seated to patient's right to enhance shadows and contouring. Inspect while patient breathes comfortably and while patient holds a deep breath. Assess symmetry, first seated at patient's side, then standing behind patient's head.	EXPECTED: Flat, rounded, or scaphoid. Contralateral areas symmetric. Maximum height of convexity at umbilicus. Abdomen remains smooth and symmetric while patient holds breath.

TECHNIQUE	FINDINGS
	UNEXPECTED: Umbilicus displaced upward, downward, or laterally or is inflamed, swollen, or bulging. Any distention (symmetric or asymmetric), bulges, or masses while breathing comfortably or holding breath.
• *Surface motion*	EXPECTED: Smooth, even motion with respiration. Female patients mostly costal movement; male patients mostly abdominal. Pulsations often visible in upper midline in thin adults. UNEXPECTED: Limited motion with respiration in male adults. Rippling movement (peristalsis) or marked pulsations.

ABDOMEN

Anatomic Correlates of the Four Quadrants of the Abdomen

Right Upper Quadrant
Liver and gallbladder
Pylorus
Duodenum
Head of pancreas
Right adrenal gland
Portion of right kidney
Hepatic flexure of colon
Portions of ascending and transverse colon

Left Upper Quadrant
Left lobe of liver
Spleen
Stomach
Body of pancreas
Left adrenal gland
Portion of left kidney
Splenic flexure of colon
Portions of transverse and descending colon

Right Lower Quadrant
Lower pole of right kidney
Cecum and appendix
Portion of ascending colon
Bladder (if distended)
Ovary and salpinx
Uterus (if enlarged)
Right spermatic cord
Right ureter

Left Lower Quadrant
Lower pole of left kidney
Sigmoid colon
Portion of descending colon
Bladder (if distended)
Ovary and salpinx
Uterus (if enlarged)
Left spermatic cord
Left ureter

ABDOMEN

TECHNIQUE	FINDINGS

Inspect abdominal muscles as patient raises head

EXPECTED: No masses or protrusions.

UNEXPECTED: Masses, protrusion of the umbilicus and other hernia signs, or separation of rectus abdominis.

Auscultate with stethoscope diaphragm

- *Frequency and character of bowel sounds*
  Warm stethoscope diaphragm, and hold with light pressure.
  May auscultate at a single site because bowel sounds generalize, but auscultate in all quadrants if you have reason to be concerned.

EXPECTED: 5 to 35 irregular clicks and gurgles per minute. Borborygmi, or increased sounds, may be because of hunger.

UNEXPECTED: Increased sounds unrelated to hunger and high-pitched tinkling sounds may be caused by early intestinal obstruction; decreased or absent sounds after 5 minutes of listening is typically associated with abdominal pain and rigidity and is a surgical emergency.

- *Liver and spleen*

EXPECTED: Silent.

UNEXPECTED: Friction rubs (high-pitched grating sound in association with respiration).

Auscultate with stethoscope bell

- *Vascular sounds*
  Listen with stethoscope bell in epigastric region, over aorta, and over renal, iliac, and femoral arteries.

EXPECTED: No bruits (harsh or musical sound indicating blood flow turbulence), venous hum (soft, low-pitched, and continuous sound), or friction rubs.

UNEXPECTED: Bruits in aortic, renal, iliac, or femoral arteries.

- *Epigastric region and around umbilicus*

EXPECTED: No venous hum.

UNEXPECTED: Venous hum.

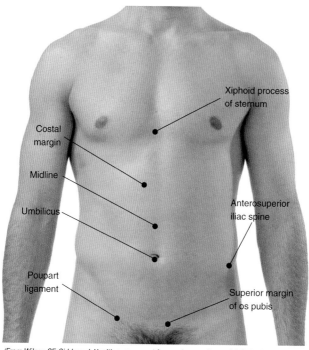

(From Wilson SF, Giddens J: Health assessment for nursing practice, ed 4, St Louis, 2009, Mosby.)

Percussion Notes of the Abdomen

NOTE	DESCRIPTION	LOCATION
Tympany	Musical note of higher pitch than resonance	Over air-filled viscera
Hyperresonance	Pitch lies between tympany and resonance	Base of left lung
Resonance	Sustained note of moderate pitch	Over lung tissue and sometimes over abdomen
Dullness	Short, high-pitched note with little resonance	Over solid organs adjacent to air-filled structures

ABDOMEN

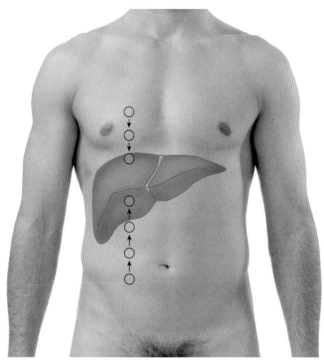

(From Wilson SF, Giddens J: Health assessment for nursing practice, ed 4, St Louis, 2009, Mosby.)

TECHNIQUE   FINDINGS

Percuss abdomen

Note: Percussion can be done independently or concurrently with palpation.

- *Tone*
  Percuss in all four
  quadrants or nine
  regions.

EXPECTED: Tympany predominant. Dullness over organs and solid masses. Dullness in suprapubic area from distended bladder. See table on p. 143 for percussion notes.
UNEXPECTED: Dullness predominant.

- *Liver span*
  To determine lower liver border, percuss upward at right midclavicular line, as shown in figure on p. 144, and mark with a pen where tympany changes to dullness. To determine upper liver border, percuss downward at right midclavicular line from an area of lung resonance, and mark change to dullness. Measure the distance between marks to estimate vertical span.

  EXPECTED: Lower border usually begins at or slightly below costal margin. Upper border usually begins at fifth to seventh intercostal space. Span generally ranges from 6 to 12 cm in adults.
  UNEXPECTED: Lower liver border >2 to 3 cm below costal margin. Upper liver border above the fifth or below the seventh intercostal space. Span <6 cm or >12 cm.

- *Spleen*
  Percuss just posterior to midaxillary line on left, beginning at areas of lung resonance and moving in several directions. Percuss lowest intercostal space in left anterior axillary line before and after patient takes deep breath.

  EXPECTED: Small area of dullness from sixth to tenth rib. Tympany before and after deep breath.
  UNEXPECTED: Large area of dullness (check for full stomach or feces-filled intestine). Tone change from tympany to dullness with inspiration.

- *Stomach*
  Percuss in area of left lower anterior rib cage and left epigastric region.

  EXPECTED: Tympany of gastric air bubble (lower than intestine tympany).
  UNEXPECTED: Dullness.

TECHNIQUE	FINDINGS
Lightly palpate abdomen	
Stand at patient's right side. Systematically palpate all quadrants, avoiding areas previously identified as problem spots. With palmar surface of fingers, depress abdominal wall up to 1 cm with light, even circular motion.	**EXPECTED:** Abdomen smooth with consistent softness. Possible tension from palpating too deeply, cold hands, or ticklishness. **UNEXPECTED:** Muscular tension or resistance, tenderness, or masses. If resistance is present, place pillow under patient's knees and ask patient to breathe slowly through mouth. Feel for relaxation of rectus abdominis muscles on expiration. Continuing tension signals involuntary response to localized or generalized rigidity.
Palpate abdomen with moderate pressure	
Using same hand position as above, palpate all quadrants again, this time with moderate pressure.	**EXPECTED:** Soft, nontender **UNEXPECTED:** Tenderness.
Deeply palpate abdomen	
With same hand position as above, repeat palpation in all quadrants or regions, pressing deeply and evenly into abdominal wall. Move fingers back and forth over abdominal contents. Use bimanual technique—exerting pressure with top hand and concentrating on sensation with bottom hand, as shown in the following figure—if obesity or muscular resistance makes deep palpation difficult. To help determine whether masses are superficial or intraabdominal, have patient lift head from examining table to contract abdominal muscles and obscure intraabdominal masses.	**EXPECTED:** Possible sensation of abdominal wall sliding back and forth. Possible awareness of borders of rectus abdominis muscles, aorta, and portions of colon. Possible tenderness over cecum, sigmoid colon, and aorta and in midline near xiphoid process. **UNEXPECTED:** Bulges, masses, tenderness unrelated to deep palpation of cecum, sigmoid colon, aorta, xiphoid process. Note location, size, shape, consistency, tenderness, pulsation, mobility, movement (with respiration) of any masses.

TECHNIQUE

FINDINGS

- *Umbilical ring and umbilicus*
  Palpate umbilical ring and around umbilicus. Note whether ring is incomplete or soft in center.

EXPECTED: Umbilical ring circular and free of irregularities. Umbilicus either slightly inverted or everted.
UNEXPECTED: Bulges, nodules, granulation. Protruding. umbilicus.

- *Liver*
  Place left hand under patient at eleventh and twelfth ribs, lifting to elevate liver toward abdominal wall. Place right hand on abdomen, fingers extended toward head with tips on right midclavicular line below level of liver dullness, as shown in figure at right. Alternatively, place right hand parallel to right costal margin, as shown in bottom figure at right. Press right hand gently but deeply in and up. Ask patient to breathe comfortably a few times and then take a deep breath. Feel for liver edge as diaphragm pushes it down. If palpable, repeat maneuver medially and laterally to costal margin.

EXPECTED: Usually liver is not palpable. If felt, liver edge should be firm, smooth, even.
UNEXPECTED: Tenderness, nodules, or irregularity.

TECHNIQUE	FINDINGS

- *Gallbladder*
  Palpate below liver margin at lateral border of rectus abdominis muscle.

  EXPECTED: Gallbladder not palpable.
  UNEXPECTED: Palpable, tender. If tender (possible cholecystitis), palpate deeply during inspiration and observe for pain (Murphy sign).

- *Spleen*
  Still standing on right side, reach across patient with left hand, place it beneath patient over left costovertebral angle (CVA), and lift spleen anteriorly toward abdominal wall. As shown in figure at right, place right hand on abdomen below left costal margin and—using findings from percussion—gently press fingertips inward toward spleen while asking patient to take a deep breath. Feel for spleen as it moves downward toward fingers.

  Repeat with patient lying on right side, as shown in bottom figure at right, with hips and knees flexed. Press inward with left hand while using fingertips of right hand to feel edge of spleen.

  EXPECTED: Spleen usually not palpable by either method.
  UNEXPECTED: Palpable spleen.

- *Left kidney*
  Standing on patient's right, reach across with left hand, and place over left flank; then place right hand at patient's left costal margin. Ask patient to inhale deeply while you elevate left flank and palpate deeply with right hand.

  EXPECTED: Left kidney usually not palpable.
  UNEXPECTED: Tenderness.

TECHNIQUE	FINDINGS
• *Right kidney* Standing on patient's right, place left hand under right flank, then place right hand at patient's right costal margin. Ask patient to inhale deeply while you elevate right flank and palpate deeply with right hand.	EXPECTED: If palpable, right kidney should be smooth and firm with rounded edges. UNEXPECTED: Tenderness.

(From Wilson SF, Giddens J: Health assessment for nursing practice, ed 4, St Louis, 2009, Mosby.)

• *Aorta* Palpate deeply slightly to left of midline and feel for aortic pulsation. As an alternative technique, place palmar surface of hands with fingers extended on midline; press fingers deeply inward on each side of aorta and feel for pulsation. For thin patients, use one hand, placing thumb and fingers on either side of aorta.	EXPECTED: If prominent, pulsation should be anterior in direction. UNEXPECTED: Prominent lateral pulsation (suggests aortic aneurysm).

• *Urinary bladder* Percuss distended bladder to help determine outline, then palpate.	EXPECTED: Ordinarily not palpable unless distended with urine. If distended, bladder should be smooth, round, and tense and on percussion will elicit lower note than surrounding air-filled intestines. UNEXPECTED: Palpable when not distended with urine.

ABDOMEN

TECHNIQUE	FINDINGS

With patient sitting, percuss CVAs

Stand behind patient. Right side: Place left hand over right CVA and strike with ulnar surface of right fist. Left side: Repeat with hands reversed.

EXPECTED: No tenderness.
UNEXPECTED: Kidney tenderness or pain.

Pain assessment

Keep eyes on patient's face while examining abdomen. To help characterize pain, have patient cough, take a deep breath, jump, or walk. Ask whether patient is hungry.

UNEXPECTED: Unwillingness to move, nausea, vomiting, areas of localized tenderness. Lack of hunger. See box and table on p. 151.

Iliopsoas muscle test

Use test for suspected appendicitis. With patient supine, place hand over right lower thigh. Ask patient to raise leg, flexing at hip, while you push downward.

UNEXPECTED: Right lower quadrant (RLQ) pain.

Obturator muscle test

Use test for suspected ruptured appendix or pelvic abscess. With patient supine, ask patient to flex right leg at hip and bend knee to 90 degrees. Hold leg just above knee, grasp ankle, and rotate leg laterally and medially, as shown in figure.

UNEXPECTED: Pain in right hypogastric region.

Some Causes of Pain Perceived in Anatomic Regions

Right Upper Quadrant
Duodenal ulcer
Hepatitis
Hepatomegaly
Lower lobe pneumonia
Cholecystitis

Right Lower Quadrant
Appendicitis
Salpingitis
Ovarian cyst
Tuboovarian abscess
Ruptured ectopic pregnancy
Renal/ureteral stone
Strangulated hernia
Meckel diverticulitis
Regional ileitis
Perforated cecum

Periumbilical
Intestinal obstruction
Acute pancreatitis
Early appendicitis

Mesenteric thrombosis
Aortic aneurysm
Diverticulitis

Left Upper Quadrant
Ruptured spleen
Gastric ulcer
Aortic aneurysm
Perforated colon
Lower lobe pneumonia

Left Lower Quadrant
Sigmoid diverticulitis
Salpingitis
Ovarian cyst
Ruptured ectopic pregnancy
Tuboovarian abscess
Renal/ureteral stone
Strangulated hernia
Perforated colon
Regional ileitis
Ulcerative colitis

Quality and Onset of Abdominal Pain

CHARACTERISTIC	POSSIBLE RELATED CONDITION
Burning	Peptic ulcer
Cramping	Biliary colic, gastroenteritis
Colic	Appendicitis with impacted feces; renal stone
Aching	Appendiceal irritation
Knifelike	Pancreatitis
Ripping, tearing	Aortic dissection
Gradual onset	Infection
Sudden onset	Duodenal ulcer, acute pancreatitis, obstruction, perforation

AIDS TO DIFFERENTIAL DIAGNOSIS

SUBJECTIVE DATA	OBJECTIVE DATA

Hiatal Hernia With Esophagitis

Epigastric pain and/or heartburn that worsens with lying down and is relieved by sitting up or antacids; water brash (mouth fills with fluid); dysphagia; sudden onset of vomiting, pain, complete dysphagia are symptoms of hernia incarceration.

Generally unremarkable exam; with severe disease, may have erythema of the posterior pharynx and edematous vocal cords.

Gastroesophageal Reflux Disease

Heartburn or acid indigestion (burning chest pain, located behind breastbone that moves up toward the neck and throat); sour taste of acid in the back of the throat or hoarseness; symptoms in infants and children include back arching or fussiness with feeding, regurgitation, and vomiting; can precipitate acute asthma exacerbation, can cause respiratory problems from aspiration, and can lead to esophageal bleeding.

Generally unremarkable exam; with severe disease, may have erythema of the posterior pharynx and edematous vocal cords; when frequent emesis occurs, may cause failure to thrive in an infant.

Duodenal Ulcer

Localized epigastric pain that occurs when the stomach is empty and is relieved with food or antacids; with upper gastrointestinal bleeding, may have hematemesis, melena, dizziness, syncope.

Anterior wall ulcers may produce tenderness on palpation of the abdomen; with significant upper gastrointestinal bleeding, may have decreased blood pressure, increased pulse rate, and decreased hematocrit level; signs of an acute abdomen could indicate perforation of duodenum, a life-threatening event.

SUBJECTIVE DATA	OBJECTIVE DATA
Acute Diarrhea	
Abrupt onset, lasts <2 weeks; abdominal pain, diarrhea, nausea, vomiting, fever, tenesmus (feeling of incomplete defecation); if symptoms occur in two or more persons after ingestion of the same food, suspect food poisoning.	Diffuse abdominal tenderness; can mimic peritoneal inflammation with RLQ pain or guarding; when severe, may develop moderate to severe dehydration (decreased blood pressure, increased heart rate).
Crohn Disease	
Chronic diarrhea (can be bloody) with malabsorption, cramping characterized by unpredictable flares and remissions.	Abdominal mass may be palpated from thickened or inflamed bowel; perianal skin tags, fistulae, and abscess formation; extraintestinal findings include arthritis of large joints, erythema nodosum, pyoderma gangrenosum.
Ulcerative Colitis	
Bloody, frequent (up to 20-30 stools/day), watery diarrhea; mild to severe symptoms based on degree of colon involvement; weight loss, fatigue, general debilitation.	Generally do not have fistulae or perianal disease; cholestatic pattern of elevated transaminases suggests sclerosing cholangitis.
Irritable Bowel Syndrome	
Cluster of symptoms consisting of abdominal pain, bloating, constipation, and diarrhea; some patients have alternating diarrhea and constipation; mucus may be present around or within the stool.	Generally unremarkable examination.
Colon Cancer	
May have abdominal pain, gross blood in stool, but more often presents with occult blood in stool on fecal occult blood test; may have change in frequency or character of stool.	With progressive disease, may have palpable mass in right (RLQ) or left lower quadrant (LLQ); rectal mass may be palpable on digital rectal examination.

ABDOMEN

SUBJECTIVE DATA	OBJECTIVE DATA
Hepatitis	
Some asymptomatic; others experience jaundice, anorexia, abdominal pain, clay-colored stools, tea-colored urine, fatigue.	Abnormal liver function tests; jaundice; hepatomegaly.
Cirrhosis	
Some asymptomatic; others experience jaundice, anorexia, abdominal pain, clay-colored stools, tea-colored urine, fatigue; may report prominent abdominal vasculature, cutaneous spider angiomas, hematemesis, abdominal fullness.	Abnormal liver function tests; jaundice; initially with firm, nontender enlarged liver; in severe disease, liver size decreases, portal hypertension and esophageal varices may develop, and muscle wasting and nutritional deficiencies may occur.
Cholecystitis	
Acute: Right upper quadrant (RUQ) pain with radiation around midtorso to right scapular region; pain is abrupt and severe, lasting 2 to 4 hours; may have fever, jaundice, anorexia. *Chronic:* Repeated acute attacks; fat intolerance, flatulence, nausea, anorexia, nonspecific abdominal pain.	Marked tenderness in the RUQ or epigastrium; involuntary guarding or rebound tenderness; some with full palpable gallbladder in RUQ.
Chronic Pancreatitis	
Unremitting abdominal pain, weight loss, steatorrhea.	Diffuse abdominal tenderness to palpation; involuntary guarding and abdominal distention can occur; elevated pancreatic enzymes (amylase and lipase); may develop pseudocyst formation; with advanced disease, may show subcutaneous fat and temporal wasting from malnutrition.

SUBJECTIVE DATA	OBJECTIVE DATA

Pyelonephritis

Flank pain, dysuria, fever; may have rigors, urinary frequency, urgency, and hematuria.

Ill appearing with CVA tenderness; pyuria and bacteria.

Renal Calculi

Fever, dysuria, hematuria; severe cramping and flank pain with nausea and vomiting; as the stone passes, pain typically moves from flank to groin to scrotal or labial area.

Ill appearing with severe cramping pain; may have CVA tenderness or abdominal tenderness on palpation; microscopic hematuria.

Appendicitis

Initially periumbilical or epigastric pain; colicky; later becomes localized to RLQ; anorexia, nausea, or vomiting after onset of pain; low-grade fever.

Guarding, tenderness, positive iliopsoas and/or obturator signs, RLQ pain on palpation (McBurney sign).

Abdominal Signs Associated With Common Abnormal Conditions

SIGN	DESCRIPTION	ASSOCIATED CONDITIONS
Aaron	Pain or distress occurs in the area of patient's heart or stomach on palpation of McBurney point	Appendicitis
Ballance	Fixed dullness to percussion in left flank and dullness in right flank that disappear on change of position	Peritoneal irritation
Blumberg	Rebound tenderness	Peritoneal irritation, appendicitis
Cullen	Ecchymosis around umbilicus	Hemoperitoneum, pancreatitis, ectopic pregnancy
Dance	Absence of bowel sounds in RLQ	Intussusception

Continued

Abdominal Signs Associated With Common Abnormal Conditions—cont'd

SIGN	DESCRIPTION	ASSOCIATED CONDITIONS
Grey Turner	Ecchymosis of flanks	Hemoperitoneum, pancreatitis
Kehr	Abdominal pain radiating to left shoulder	Spleen rupture, renal calculi, ectopic pregnancy
Markle (heel jar)	Patient stands with straightened knees, then raises up on toes, relaxes, and allows heels to hit floor, thus jarring body; action will cause abdominal pain if positive	Peritoneal irritation, appendicitis
McBurney	Rebound tenderness and sharp pain when McBurney point is palpated (⅔ the distance from the umbilicus to the anterior superior iliac spine)	Appendicitis
Murphy	Abrupt cessation of inspiration on palpation of gallbladder	Cholecystitis
Romberg-Howship	Pain down medial aspect of thigh to knees	Strangulated obturator hernia
Rovsing	RLQ pain intensified by left lower quadrant abdominal palpation	Peritoneal irritation, appendicitis

Conditions Producing Acute Abdominal Pain

CONDITION	USUAL PAIN CHARACTERISTICS	POSSIBLE ASSOCIATED FINDINGS
Appendicitis	Initially periumbilical or epigastric; colicky; later becomes localized to RLQ, often at McBurney point	Guarding, tenderness; positive iliopsoas and positive obturator tests, RLQ skin hyperesthesia; anorexia, nausea, or vomiting after onset of pain; low-grade fever; positive Aaron, Rovsing, Markle, and McBurney signs*
Peritonitis	Onset sudden or gradual; pain generalized or localized, dull or severe and unrelenting; guarding; pain on deep inspiration	Shallow respiration; positive Blumberg, Markle, and Ballance signs; reduced bowel sounds, nausea and vomiting; positive obturator and iliopsoas tests

ABDOMEN

Conditions Producing Acute Abdominal Pain—cont'd

CONDITION	USUAL PAIN CHARACTERISTICS	POSSIBLE ASSOCIATED FINDINGS
Cholecystitis	Severe, unrelenting RUQ or epigastric pain; may be referred to right subscapular area	RUQ tenderness and rigidity, positive Murphy sign, palpable gallbladder, anorexia, vomiting, fever, possible jaundice
Pancreatitis	Dramatic, sudden, excruciating left upper quadrant (LUQ), epigastric, or umbilical pain; may be present in one or both flanks; may be referred to left shoulder	Epigastric tenderness, vomiting, fever, shock; positive Grey Turner sign; positive Cullen sign; both signs may occur 2 to 3 days after onset
Salpingitis	Lower quadrant, worse on left	Nausea, vomiting, fever, suprapubic tenderness, rigid abdomen, pain on pelvic examination
Pelvic inflammatory disease	Lower quadrant, increases with activity	Tender adnexa and cervix, cervical discharge, dyspareunia
Diverticulitis	Epigastric, radiating down left side of abdomen especially after eating; may be referred to back	Flatulence, borborygmi, diarrhea, dysuria, tenderness on palpation
Perforated gastric or duodenal ulcer	Abrupt RUQ; may be referred to shoulders	Abdominal free air and distention with increased resonance over liver; tenderness in epigastrium or RUQ; rigid abdominal wall, rebound tenderness
Intestinal obstruction	Abrupt, severe, spasmodic; referred to epigastrium, umbilicus	Distention, minimal rebound tenderness, vomiting, localized tenderness, visible peristalsis; bowel sounds absent (with paralytic obstruction) or hyperactive high-pitched (with mechanical obstruction)
Volvulus	Referred to hypogastrium and umbilicus	Distention, nausea, vomiting, guarding; sigmoid loop volvulus may be palpable
Leaking abdominal aneurysm	Steady throbbing midline over aneurysm; may penetrate to back, flank	Nausea, vomiting, abdominal mass, bruit

ABDOMEN

Continued

Conditions Producing Acute Abdominal Pain—cont'd

CONDITION	USUAL PAIN CHARACTERISTICS	POSSIBLE ASSOCIATED FINDINGS
Biliary stones, colic	Episodic, severe, RUQ, or epigastrium lasting 15 minutes to several hours; may be referred to subscapular area, especially right	RUQ tenderness, soft abdominal wall, anorexia, vomiting, jaundice, subnormal temperature
Renal calculi	Intense; flank, extending to groin and genitals; may be episodic	Fever, hematuria; positive Kehr sign
Ectopic pregnancy	Lower quadrant; referred to shoulder; with rupture is agonizing	Hypogastric tenderness, symptoms of pregnancy, spotting, irregular menses, soft abdominal wall, mass on bimanual pelvic examination; ruptured: shock, rigid abdominal wall, distention; positive Kehr, Cullen signs
Ruptured ovarian cyst	Lower quadrant, steady, increases with cough or motion	Vomiting, low-grade fever, anorexia, tenderness on pelvic examination
Splenic rupture	Intense; LUQ, radiating to left shoulder; may worsen with foot of bed elevated	Shock, pallor, lowered temperature

*See table on pp. 155-156 for explanation of signs.

Conditions Producing Chronic Abdominal Pain

CONDITION	USUAL PAIN CHARACTERISTICS	POSSIBLE ASSOCIATED FINDINGS
Irritable bowel syndrome	Hypogastric pain; crampy, variable, infrequent; associated with bowel function	Unremarkable physical examination; pain associated with gas, bloating, distention; relief with passage of flatus, feces
Lactose intolerance	Crampy pain after drinking milk or eating milk products	Associated diarrhea; unremarkable physical examination
Diverticular disease	Localized pain	Abdominal tenderness, fever

Conditions Producing Chronic Abdominal Pain—cont'd

CONDITION	USUAL PAIN CHARACTERISTICS	POSSIBLE ASSOCIATED FINDINGS
Constipation	Colicky or dull and steady pain that does not progress or worsen	Fecal mass palpable, stool in rectum
Uterine fibroids	Pain related to menses, intercourse	Palpable myoma(s)
Hernia	Localized pain that increases with exertion or lifting	Hernia on physical examination
Esophagitis/gastroesophageal reflux disease	Burning, gnawing pain in midepigastrium, worsens with recumbency	Unremarkable physical examination
Peptic ulcer	Burning or gnawing pain	May have epigastric tenderness on palpation
Gastritis	Constant burning pain in epigastrium	May be accompanied by nausea, vomiting, diarrhea, or fever; unremarkable physical examination

Modified from Dains JE, Baumann LC, Dains PS: *Advanced health assessment & clinical diagnosis in primary care,* St. Louis: Mosby, 2011.

Differential Diagnosis of Urinary Incontinence

CONDITION	HISTORY	PHYSICAL FINDINGS
Stress incontinence	Small-volume incontinence with coughing, sneezing, laughing, running; history of prior pelvic surgery	Pelvic floor relaxation; cystocele, rectocele; lax urethral sphincter; loss of urine with provocative testing; atrophic vaginitis; postvoid residual <100 mL
Urge incontinence	Uncontrolled urge to void; large-volume incontinence; history of central nervous system disorders such as stroke, multiple sclerosis, parkinsonism	Unexpected findings only as related to central nervous system disorder; postvoid residual <100 mL

Continued

ABDOMEN

Differential Diagnosis of Urinary Incontinence—cont'd

CONDITION	HISTORY	PHYSICAL FINDINGS
Overflow incontinence	Small-volume incontinence, dribbling, hesitancy; in men, symptoms of enlarged prostate: nocturia, dribbling, hesitancy, decreased force and caliber of stream	Distended bladder; prostate hypertrophy; stool in rectum, fecal impaction; postvoid residual >100 mL
	In neurogenic bladder: history of bowel problems, spinal cord injury, or multiple sclerosis	Evidence of spinal cord disease or diabetic neuropathy; lax sphincter; gait disturbance
Functional incontinence	Change in mental status, impaired mobility, new environment	Impaired mental status; impaired mobility
	Medications: hypnotics, diuretics, anticholinergic agents, α-adrenergic agents, calcium channel blockers	Impaired mental status or unexpected findings only as related to other physical conditions

PEDIATRIC VARIATIONS

EXAMINATION

TECHNIQUE	FINDINGS

Inspect abdomen in all four quadrants

Infant's abdomen should be examined, if possible, during a time of relaxation and quiet. Sucking on a pacifier may help to relax infant. The parent's lap can serve as the best examining surface for toddlers through age 2 to 3 years.

- *Contour/ symmetry*

  EXPECTED: Until the age of 3 years, abdomen will protrude when standing.

  UNEXPECTED: Distention can indicate organ enlargement, fecal impaction, or abdominal mass.

- *Surface motion*

  EXPECTED: Pulsation in epigastric area in newborns and infants.

  UNEXPECTED: Peristaltic waves associated with pyloric stenosis.

TECHNIQUE	FINDINGS

Percuss abdomen

- *Tone* EXPECTED: More tympany is present in infants than adults because of air swallowing during crying and feeding.

Lightly and deeply palpate abdomen

- *Umbilical ring* EXPECTED: Infants and children may have an umbilical hernia (typically closes spontaneously by 1-2 years of age).
- *Liver* EXPECTED: Liver may be palpable in young children 2 to 3 cm below costal margin.

Age	Liver Span (cm)
6 mo	2.4 to 2.8
12 mo	2.8 to 3.1
24 mo	3.5 to 3.6
3 yr	4.0
4 yr	4.3 to 4.4
5 yr	4.5 to 5.1
6 yr	4.8 to 5.1
8 yr	5.1 to 5.6
10 yr	5.5 to 6.1

Sample Documentation

Subjective. A 44-year-old woman describes a burning sensation in the epigastric area and chest. Occurs after eating, especially with spicy foods. Lasts 1 to 2 hours and is worse when lying down. Sometimes causes bitter taste in mouth. Also feels bloated. Antacids do not relieve symptoms. Denies nausea/vomiting/diarrhea. No cough or shortness of breath.

Objective. Abdomen rounded and symmetric, with white striae adjacent to umbilicus in all quadrants. A well-healed, 5-cm, white surgical scar evident in RLQ. No areas of visible pulsations or peristalsis. Active bowel sounds audible. Percussion tones tympanic over epigastrium. Liver span 8 cm at right midclavicular line. On inspiration, liver edge firm, smooth, and nontender. No splenomegaly. Musculature soft and relaxed to light palpation. No masses or areas of tenderness to deep palpation. No CVA tenderness.

15 Female Genitalia

Equipment

- Lamp or light source
- Drapes
- Speculum
- Gloves
- Water-soluble lubricant
- Papanicolaou (Pap) smear/human papillomavirus (HPV) collection equipment:
    - Collection device (wooden or plastic spatula; cervical brush or broom)
    - Glass slides and cytologic fixative or fluid collection media
- Other specimen collection equipment as needed:
    - Cotton swabs
    - Culture plates or media
    - DNA tests for organisms

EXAMINATION

Have patient in lithotomy position, draped for minimal exposure.

FEMALE GENITALIA

TECHNIQUE	FINDINGS

External Genitalia

Wash or sanitize hands and wear gloves on both hands

Ask patient to separate or drop open the knees. Tell patient you are beginning the examination, then touch lower thigh and—without breaking contact—move hand along thigh to external genitalia.

Inspect and palpate mons pubis

• *Characteristics*	EXPECTED: Skin smooth and clean. UNEXPECTED: Improper hygiene.
• *Pubic hair*	EXPECTED: Female pattern distribution. UNEXPECTED: Nits or lice.

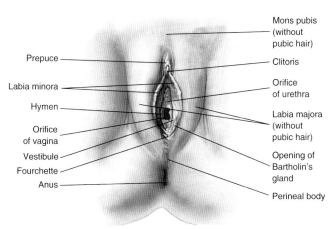

Mons pubis (without pubic hair)

Prepuce

Clitoris

Labia minora

Orifice of urethra

Hymen

Orifice of vagina

Labia majora (without pubic hair)

Vestibule

Fourchette

Opening of Bartholin's gland

Anus

Perineal body

(From Lowdermilk DL, Perry SE: Maternity and women's health care, ed 8, St Louis, 2007, Mosby.)

Inspect and palpate labia

• *Labia majora*	EXPECTED: Gaping or closed, dry or moist, shriveled or full, tissue soft and homogeneous, usually symmetric.

TECHNIQUE	FINDINGS
	UNEXPECTED: Swelling, redness, tenderness, discoloration, varicosities, obvious stretching, or signs of trauma or scarring. If excoriation, rashes, or lesions are present, ask patient about scratching
• *Labia minora* Separate labia majora with fingers of one hand. With other hand, palpate labia minora between thumb and second finger.	**EXPECTED:** Moist, dark pink inner surface. Tissue soft and homogeneous. **UNEXPECTED:** Tenderness, inflammation, irritation, excoriation, caking of discharge in tissue folds, discoloration, ulcers, vesicles, irregularities, or nodules. Hyperemia of fourchette not related to recent sexual activity.

Inspect clitoris

• *Size and length*	**EXPECTED:** Length ≤2 cm; diameter 0.5 cm. **UNEXPECTED:** Enlargement, atrophy, inflammation, or adhesions.

Inspect urethral meatus and vaginal opening

• *Urethral orifice*	**EXPECTED:** Slit or irregular opening, close to or in vaginal introitus, usually midline. **UNEXPECTED:** Discharge, polyps, caruncles, fistulas, lesions, irritation, inflammation, or dilation.
• *Vaginal introitus*	**EXPECTED:** Thin vertical slit or large orifice with irregular edges. Tissue moist. **UNEXPECTED:** Swelling, discoloration, discharge, lesions, fistulas, or fissures.

TECHNIQUE	FINDINGS

Milk Skene glands

Tell patient you will be inserting one finger into the vagina and pressing forward with it. With palm up, insert index finger to second joint, press upward, and milk Skene glands by moving finger outward. Perform on both sides of urethra and directly on urethra.

UNEXPECTED: Discharge or tenderness. Note color, consistency, odor of any discharge; obtain culture.

Palpate Bartholin glands

Tell patient to expect to feel you pressing around the entrance to the vagina. Palpate lateral tissue between index finger and thumb, then palpate entire area bilaterally, particularly postero-lateral portion of labia majora.

EXPECTED: No swelling.
UNEXPECTED: Swelling, tenderness, masses, heat, fluctuation, or discharge. Note color, consistency, odor of any discharge; obtain culture.

Test vaginal muscle tone if indicated

Ask patient to squeeze vaginal opening around your finger.

EXPECTED: Fairly tight squeezing by some nulliparous patients, less so by some multiparous patients.
UNEXPECTED: Protrusion of cervix or uterus.

Locate the cervix

With your finger still in place, reach in farther to locate the cervix and note the direction in which it points. This may help you locate the cervix when you insert the speculum.

EXPECTED: Midline, may point horizontally, anteriorly, or posteriorly.
UNEXPECTED: Deviates to right or left.

TECHNIQUE	FINDINGS

Inspect for bulging and urinary incontinence if indicated

Ask patient to bear down.

EXPECTED: No bulging.
UNEXPECTED: Bulging of anterior or posterior wall, or urinary incontinence.

Inspect and palpate perineum

Compress perineal tissue between finger and thumb.

EXPECTED: Perineum surface smooth—generally thick and smooth in a nulliparous patient, thinner and rigid in a multiparous patient. Possible episiotomy scarring from childbirth.
UNEXPECTED: Tenderness, inflammation, fistulas, lesions, or growths.

Inspect anus

• *Skin characteristics*

EXPECTED: Skin darkly pigmented and possibly coarse.
UNEXPECTED: Scarring, lesions, inflammation, fissures, lumps, skin tags, or excoriation.

Internal Genitalia—Speculum Examination

If you touched the perineum or anal skin while examining the external genitalia, change gloves before beginning internal examination. Lubricate speculum and gloved fingers with water or water-soluble gel lubricant. Water is preferred if obtaining a Pap smear.

Insert speculum

Tell patient you will be touching again; then insert two fingers of hand not holding the speculum just inside vaginal introitus and gently press downward. Ask patient to breathe slowly and try to consciously relax pelvic and buttock muscles.

FEMALE GENITALIA

TECHNIQUE	FINDINGS

Use fingers of that hand to separate labia minora widely so that
the vaginal opening becomes
clearly visible. Then slowly insert
speculum along path of least
resistance, often slightly downward, avoiding trauma to urethra
and vaginal walls. Some clinicians insert speculum blades at
an oblique angle; others prefer
to keep blades horizontal.
Avoid touching clitoris, catching
pubic hair, or pinching labial
skin. Insert speculum the length
of the vaginal canal. Maintaining downward pressure, open
speculum by pressing on thumb
piece. Sweep speculum slowly
upward until cervix comes into
view. Adjust light, then ma-
nipulate speculum farther into
vagina to fully expose the cervix
between anterior and posterior
blades. Stabilize distal spread
of blades and adjust proximal
spread as needed.

Inspect cervix

• *Color*

*(From Edge V, Miller M: Women's health care,
St Louis, 1994, Mosby.)*

EXPECTED: Evenly distributed
pink. Symmetric, circum-
scribed erythema around os
can be expected.
UNEXPECTED: Bluish, pale, or
reddened cervix (especially
if patchy or with irregular
borders).

FEMALE GENITALIA

TECHNIQUE	FINDINGS
• *Position*	EXPECTED: In midline, horizontal, or pointing anteriorly or posteriorly. Protruding into vagina 1 to 3 cm. UNEXPECTED: Deviation to right or left. Protrusion into vagina >1 to 3 cm.
• *Size*	EXPECTED: 3 cm in diameter. UNEXPECTED: >3 cm.
• *Shape*	EXPECTED: Uniform. UNEXPECTED: Distorted.
• *Surface characteristics*	EXPECTED: Surface smooth. Possible symmetric, reddened circle around os (squamocolumnar epithelium). Possible small, white, or yellow raised round areas on cervix (nabothian cysts). UNEXPECTED: Friable tissue, red patchy areas, granular areas, or white patches.
• *Discharge* Note any discharge. Determine origin—cervix or vagina.	EXPECTED: Odorless; creamy or clear; thick, thin, or stringy (often heavier at midcycle or immediately before menstruation). UNEXPECTED: Odorous and white to yellow, green, or gray.
• *Size and shape of os* Follow standard precautions for safe collection of human secretions.	EXPECTED: Nulliparous patient: small, round, oval. Multiparous patient: usually a horizontal slit or irregular and stellate. UNEXPECTED: Slit resulting from trauma from induced abortion, difficult removal of intrauterine device, or sexual abuse.

FEMALE GENITALIA

TECHNIQUE	FINDINGS

Withdraw speculum and inspect vaginal walls

Unlock speculum and re-move it slowly, rotating it so vaginal walls can be inspected. Maintain downward pressure and hook index finger over anterior blade as it is removed. Note odor of any discharge pooled in posterior blade, and obtain specimen if not already obtained.

EXPECTED: Vaginal wall color same pink as cervix or lighter; moist, smooth or rugated; and homogeneous. Thin, clear or cloudy, odorless secretions. UNEXPECTED: Reddened patches, lesions, pallor, cracks, bleeding, nodules, swelling. Se-cretions that are profuse; thick, curdy, or frothy; gray, green, or yellow; or malodorous.

Internal Genitalia—Bimanual Examination

Change gloves, then lubricate index and middle fingers of examining hand.
Tell patient you are going to examine internally with your fingers.
Prevent thumb from touching clitoris during examination.

Obtaining Vaginal Smears and Cultures

Vaginal specimens for smears and cultures are often obtained during the speculum examination. Vaginal specimens are obtained while the speculum is in place but after the cervix and its surrounding tissue have been inspected. Collect specimens as indicated for Pap smear, HPV testing, sexually transmit-ted infection screening, and wet mount. Be sure to follow Standard Precau-tions for the safe collection of human secretions. Label the specimen with the patient's name, date, and a description of the specimen (e.g., cervical smear, vaginal smear, culture). If the Pap smear cervical specimen is from a transgender man, it is essential to make clear to the laboratory that the sample is a cervical Pap smear (especially if the listed gender marker is "male") to avoid the sample being run incorrectly as an anal Pap smear or discarded. The use of testosterone or the presence of amenorrhea should be indicated on the requisition.

Conventional Pap Smear
Brushes and brooms are now being used in conjunction with or instead of the conventional spatula to improve the quality of cells obtained. The cylindric-type brush (e.g., a Cytobrush) collects endocervical cells only. First, collect a sample

Continued

from the ectocervix with a spatula. Insert the longer projection of the spatula into the cervical os. Rotate it 360 degrees, keeping it flush against the cervical tissue. Withdraw the spatula, and spread the specimen on a glass slide. A single light stroke with each side of the spatula is sufficient to thin out the specimen over the slide. Fix the specimen, and label as ectocervical. Then introduce the brush device into the vagina, and insert it into the cervical os until only the bristles closest to the handle are exposed. Slowly rotate one-half to one full turn. Remove it, and prepare the slide. A single light stroke with each side of the spatula is sufficient to thin out the specimen over the slide. Fix the specimen, and label it as ectocervical. Then introduce the brush device into the vagina, and insert it into the cervical os until only the bristles closest to the handle are exposed. Slowly rotate one-half to one full turn. Remove it, and prepare the endocervical smear by rolling the brush with moderate pressure across a glass slide. Fix the specimen, and label it as endocervical. Alternatively, both specimens can be placed on a single slide.

The broom-type brush is used for collecting ectocervical and endocervical cells at the same time. The broom has flexible plastic bristles, which are reported to cause less blood spotting after the examination. Introduce the brush into the vagina, and insert the central long bristles into the cervical os until the lateral bristles bend fully against the ectocervix. Maintain gentle pressure, and rotate the brush by rolling the handle between the thumb and forefinger three to five times to the left and right. Withdraw the brush, and transfer the sample to a glass slide with two single "paint" strokes. Apply first one side of the bristle, then turn the brush over and paint the slide again in exactly the same area. Apply fixative, and label the specimen as ectocervical and endocervical.

Liquid Based Testing

The liquid-based cytology replaces the use of a glass slide and fixative spray. Use a brush and/or the broom-type device to collect the specimen, following the same collection steps as with the conventional Pap smear. Rinse the brush in the solution by swirling. Deposit the broom end of the device directly into the collection vial. With any collection device, be sure to follow the manufacturer's and laboratory instructions to collect and preserve the specimen appropriately. Close the vial tightly to prevent leakage and loss of the sample during transport. Label it with the patient's name, the date, and the origin of the specimen (ectocervical only or ectocervical and endocervical). The liquid sample is also used to test for HPV.

Gonococcal Culture Specimen

Immediately after the Pap smear is obtained, introduce a sterile cotton swab into the vagina and insert it into the cervical os. Hold it in place for 10 to 30 seconds. Withdraw the swab and spread the specimen in a large z pattern over the culture medium, rotating the swab at the same time. Label the tube or plate, and follow agency routine for transporting and warming the specimen. If indicated, an anal culture can be obtained after the vaginal speculum has been removed. Insert a fresh, sterile cotton swab about 2.5 cm into the rectum, and rotate it in a full circle. Hold it in place for 10 to 30 seconds. Withdraw the swab, and prepare the specimen as described for the vaginal culture. Gonococcal cultures are now used less frequently than DNA testing for chlamydia and gonorrhea.

(From Grimes D: Infectious diseases, St Louis, 1991, Mosby.)

DNA Testing for Organisms

Use a Dacron swab (with a plastic or wire shaft) when collecting the specimen; wooden, cotton-tipped applicators may interfere with test results. Also be sure to check the expiration date so as not to use out-of-date materials. Insert the swab into the cervical os, and rotate the swab in the endocervical canal for 30 seconds to ensure adequate sampling and absorption by the swab. Avoid contact with the vaginal mucous membranes, which would contaminate the specimen. Remove the swab and place it in the tube containing the specimen reagent. Single- or dual-organism tests are available for *Chlamydia trachomatis* and *Neisseria gonorrhoeae.* Multiorganism tests are available for *Trichomonas vaginalis, Gardnerella vaginalis,* and *Candida* species

Wet Mount and Potassium Hydroxide Procedures

In a patient with vaginal discharge, these microscope examinations can demonstrate the presence of *T. vaginalis,* bacterial vaginosis, or candidiasis. For the wet mount, obtain a specimen of vaginal discharge using a swab. Smear the sample on a glass slide, and add a drop of normal saline solution. Place a coverslip on the slide and view under the microscope. The presence of trichomonads indicates *T. vaginalis.* The presence of bacteria-filled epithelial cells (clue cells) indicates bacterial vaginosis. On a separate glass slide, place a specimen of vaginal discharge, apply a drop of aqueous 10% potassium hydroxide (KOH), and put a coverslip in place. The presence of a fishy odor (the "whiff test") suggests bacterial vaginosis. The KOH dissolves epithelial cells and debris and facilitates visualization of the mycelia of a fungus. View the specimen under the microscope for the presence of mycelial fragments, hyphae, and budding yeast cells, which indicate candidiasis.

TECHNIQUE	FINDINGS

Palpate vaginal wall while inserting fingers into vagina

Insert tips of index and middle fingers into vaginal opening and press downward, waiting for muscles to relax. Gradually insert fingers full length while palpating vaginal wall.

EXPECTED: Smooth and homogeneous.
UNEXPECTED: Tenderness, lesions, cysts, nodules, masses, or growths.

Palpate cervix

Locate cervix with palmar surface of fingers, feel end, and run fingers around circumference to feel fornices.

- *Size, shape, length*

  EXPECTED: Consistent with speculum examination.

- *Consistency*

  EXPECTED: Firm in non-pregnant patient; softer in pregnant patient.
  UNEXPECTED: Nodules, hardness, or roughness.

- *Position*

  EXPECTED: In midline horizontal or pointing anteriorly or posteriorly. Protruding into vagina 1 to 3 cm.
  UNEXPECTED: Deviation to right or left. Protrusion into vagina >1 to 3 cm.

- *Mobility*

  Grasp cervix gently between fingers and move from side to side. Observe patient's facial expression.

  EXPECTED: 1- to 2-cm movement in each direction. Minimal discomfort.
  UNEXPECTED: Pain on movement ("cervical motion tenderness").

TECHNIQUE

FINDINGS

Palpate uterus

• *Location and position*
Place palmar surface of
outside hand on abdominal
midline, halfway between
umbilicus and symphysis
pubis, and place intravaginal
fingers in anterior fornix.
Slowly slide outside hand
toward pubis while press-
ing down and forward with
flat surface of fingers; at
the same time, push inward
and up with fingertips of
intravaginal hand while
pushing down on cervix with
backs of fingers. If uterus is
anteverted or anteflexed, you
should feel fundus between
fingers of two hands at level
of pubis. If uterus cannot
be felt with this maneuver,
place intravaginal fingers
together in posterior fornix
and outside hand immedi-
ately above symphysis pubis.
Press down firmly with
outside hand while pressing
inward against cervix with
intravaginal hand. If uterus
is retroverted or retroflexed,
you should feel fundus. If
uterus cannot be felt with
either of these maneuvers,
move intravaginal fingers to
each side of cervix, and while
keeping contact with cervix,
press inward and feel as far
as possible.

EXPECTED: In midline, horizontal, or pointing anteriorly
or posteriorly. Protruding into
vagina 1 to 3 cm.
UNEXPECTED: Deviation to
right or left. Protrusion into
vagina >1 to 3 cm.

TECHNIQUE

FINDINGS

Slide fingers so they are on top and bottom of cervix, and continue pressing in while moving fingers to feel as much of uterus as possible (when uterus is in midposition, you will not be able to feel it with outside hand).

A

B

C

D   E

A, Retroverted. *B,* Anteflexed. *C,* Anteverted. *D,* Midline. *E,* Retroflexed.

• *Size, shape, contour*	EXPECTED: Pear-shaped and 5.5 to 8 cm long (larger in all dimensions in multiparous patients). Contour rounded and, in nonpregnant patients, walls firm and smooth. UNEXPECTED: Larger than expected or interrupted contour or smoothness.
• *Mobility* Gently move uterus between intravaginal fingers and outside hand.	EXPECTED: Mobile in anteroposterior plane. UNEXPECTED: Fixed uterus or tenderness on movement.

Palpate ovaries

Place fingers of outside hand on lower right quadrant. With intravaginal hand facing up, place both fingers in right lateral fornix. Press intravaginal fingers deeply in and up toward abdominal hand, while sweeping flat surface of fingers of outside hand deeply in and obliquely down toward symphysis pubis. Palpate entire area by firmly pressing outside hand and intravaginal fingers together. Repeat on left side.

TECHNIQUE	FINDINGS
• *Consistency*	EXPECTED: If palpable, ovaries should feel firm, smooth, slightly to moderately tender. UNEXPECTED: Marked tenderness or nodularity. Palpable fallopian tubes.
• *Size*	EXPECTED: About 3 × 2 × 1 cm. UNEXPECTED: Enlargement.
• *Shape*	EXPECTED: Ovoid. UNEXPECTED: Distorted.

Palpate adnexal areas

Use hand positions for palpating ovaries.

EXPECTED: Adnexa difficult to palpate.
UNEXPECTED: Masses and tenderness. If adnexal masses are found, characterize by size, shape, location, consistency, tenderness.

Internal Genitalia—Rectovaginal Examination

Change gloves. This examination may be uncomfortable for the patient. Assure that the urgent feeling of a bowel movement will pass. Ask the patient to breathe slowly and try to relax the sphincter, rectum, and buttocks.

Insert index finger into vagina and middle finger into anus

To insert middle finger into anus, press against anus and ask patient to bear down; slip tip of finger into rectum just past sphincter.

Assess sphincter tone

Palpate area of anorectal junction and just above it. Ask patient to tighten and relax anal sphincter.

EXPECTED: Even sphincter tightening.
UNEXPECTED: Extremely tight, lax, or absent sphincter.

TECHNIQUE	FINDINGS

Palpate anterior rectal wall and rectovaginal septum

Slide both fingers in as far as possible, then ask patient to bear down. Rotate rectal finger to explore anterior rectal wall and palpate rectovaginal septum.

EXPECTED: Smooth and uninterrupted. Uterine body and uterine fundus sometimes felt with retroflexed uterus.
UNEXPECTED: Masses, polyps, nodules, strictures, irregularities, tenderness.

Palpate posterior aspect of uterus

Place outside hand just above symphysis pubis and press firmly and deeply down, while positioning intravaginal finger in posterior vaginal fornix and pressing strongly upward against posterior side of cervix, as shown in the following figure. Palpate as much of posterior side of uterus as possible.

EXPECTED: Consistent with bimanual examination regarding location, position, size, shape, contour.
UNEXPECTED: Tenderness.

(From Lowdermilk DL, Perry SE: Maternity and women's health care, ed 8, St Louis, 2007, Mosby.)

FEMALE GENITALIA

TECHNIQUE	FINDINGS
Palpate posterior rectal wall	
As you withdraw fingers, rotate intrarectal finger to evaluate posterior rectal wall.	EXPECTED: Smooth and uninterrupted. UNEXPECTED: Masses, polyps, nodules, strictures, irregularities, tenderness.
Note characteristics of feces when gloved finger removed	
	EXPECTED: Light to dark brown. UNEXPECTED: Blood. Note color and prepare specimen for fecal occult blood test if indicated.
Unless unable to, let patient wipe off the lubricating gel	

AIDS TO DIFFERENTIAL DIAGNOSIS

SUBJECTIVE DATA	OBJECTIVE DATA
Premenstrual Syndrome	
Breast swelling and tenderness, acne, bloating and weight gain, headache or joint pain, food cravings, irritability, difficulty concentrating, mood swings, crying spells, depression. Symptoms occur 5 to 7 days before menses (luteal phase) and subside with onset of menses.	None; diagnosis based on symptoms.
Endometriosis	
Pelvic pain, dysmenorrhea, heavy or prolonged menstrual flow.	May have no physical findings; on bimanual examination, tender nodules may be palpable along the uterosacral ligaments. Diagnosis confirmed by laparoscopy.

SUBJECTIVE DATA	OBJECTIVE DATA
Condylomata Acuminata (Genital Warts)	
Warty lesions on labia, within vestibule, or in perianal region.	Flesh-colored, whitish pink to reddish brown, discrete, soft growths on labia, vestibule, or perianal area; may occur singly or in clusters and may enlarge to cauliflower masses.
Genital Herpes	
Painful lesions in genital area; history of sexual contact; may report burning or pain with urination.	Small, red vesicles in genital area.
Vaginal Infections	
Vaginal discharge, possibly accompanied by urinary symptoms. Sometimes asymptomatic.	See table on pp. 181-182.
Cervical Carcinoma	
Often asymptomatic; sometimes vaginal bleeding.	Hard, granular surface at or near cervical os. Lesion can evolve to form extensive, irregular, easily bleeding cauliflower growth. Precancerous and early cancer changes detected by Pap smear, not by physical examination.

Uterine Bleeding

See table on p. 183. Terminology:

- Amenorrhea: absence of menstruation
- Polymenorrhea: shortened interval between periods—<19 to 21 days
- Oligomenorrhea: lengthened interval between periods—>35 days

SUBJECTIVE DATA	OBJECTIVE DATA
• Hypermenorrhea: excessive flow during normal duration of regular periods • Hypomenorrhea: decreased flow during normal duration of regular periods • Menorrhagia: regular and normal interval between periods, excessive flow and duration • Metrorrhagia: irregular interval between periods, excessive flow and duration • Menometrorrhagia: irregular or excessive bleeding during periods and between periods	

Pelvic Inflammatory Disease (PID)

Painful intercourse, painful urination, irregular menstrual bleeding, pain in the right upper abdomen.	*Acute PID:* Very tender bilateral adnexal areas. *Chronic PID:* Bilateral tender, irregular, fairly fixed adnexal areas.

Ovarian Cancer

Persistent and unexplained vague gastrointestinal symptoms such as generalized abdominal discomfort and/or pain, gas, indigestion, pressure, swelling, bloating, cramps, or feeling of fullness even after a light meal.	May have no physical findings; on bimanual examination, an enlarged ovary in premenopausal patient or a palpable ovary in postmenopausal patients.

Differential Diagnosis of Vaginal Discharges and Infections

CONDITION	HISTORY	PHYSICAL FINDINGS	DIAGNOSTIC TESTS
Physiologic vaginitis	Increase in discharge; no foul odor, itching, or edema	Clear or mucoid discharge; pH <4.5	Wet mount: up to 3 to 5 white blood cells (WBCs); epithelial cells
Bacterial vaginosis (G. vaginalis)	Foul-smelling discharge; has concern about "fishy odor"	Homogeneous, thin, white or gray discharge; pH ≥4.5	Positive KOH "whiff" test; wet mount: positive clue cells
Candida vulvovaginitis (Candida albicans)	Pruritic discharge, itching of labia; itching may extend to thighs	White, curdy discharge; pH 4.0 to 5.0; cervix may be red; may have erythema of perineum and thighs	KOH prep: Mycelia, budding, branching yeast, pseudo-hyphae
Trichomoniasis (T. vaginalis)	Watery discharge; foul odor; dysuria and dyspareunia with severe infection	Profuse, frothy, greenish discharge; pH 5.0 to 6.6; red friable cervix with petechiae ("strawberry" cervix)	Wet mount: Round or pear-shaped protozoa, motile "gyrating" flagella
Gonorrhea (N. gonorrhoeae)	Partner with sexually transmitted disease; often asymptomatic or may have symptoms of pelvic inflammatory disease (PID)	Purulent discharge from cervix; Skene/Bartholin gland inflam-mation; cervix and vulva may be inflamed	Gram stain, culture, DNA probe
Chlamydia (C. trachomatis)	Partner with nongonococcal urethritis; often asymptomatic; may express concern about spotting after intercourse or urethritis	With or without purulent discharge; cervix may or may not be red or friable	DNA probe

Atrophic vaginitis   Dyspareunia; vaginal dryness; perimeno-   Pale, thin vaginal mucosa; pH >4.5   Wet mount: Folded, clumped
                      pausal or postmenopausal   epithelial cells

Allergic vaginitis   New bubble bath, soap, douche, or other   Foul smell, erythema; pH <4.5   Wet mount: WBCs
                      hygiene products

Foreign body   Red and swollen vulva; vaginal dis-   Bloody or foul-smelling discharge   Wet mount: WBCs
                      charge; history of tampon, condom, or
                      diaphragm use

Bacterial vaginosis   Candida vulvovaginitis   Trichomoniasis

Types of Uterine Bleeding and Associated Causes

TYPE	COMMON CAUSES
Midcycle spotting	Midcycle estradiol fluctuation associated with ovulation
Delayed menstruation	Anovulation or threatened abortion with excessive bleeding
Frequent bleeding	Chronic pelvic inflammatory disease (PID), endometriosis, dysfunctional uterine bleeding (DUB), anovulation
Profuse menstrual bleeding	Endometrial polyps, DUB, adenomyosis, submucous leiomyomas, intrauterine device
Intermenstrual or irregular bleeding	Endometrial polyps, DUB, uterine or cervical cancer, oral contraceptives
Postmenopausal bleeding	Endometrial hyperplasia, estrogen therapy, endometrial cancer

PEDIATRIC VARIATIONS

EXAMINATION

TECHNIQUE	FINDINGS

Inspect external genitalia

Examine infant using the frog-leg position.

EXPECTED: Genitalia of newborn reflect influence of maternal hormones. Labia majora and minora may be swollen, with labia minora often more prominent.

Inspect clitoris

* *Size and length*

EXPECTED: The clitoris of a term infant is usually covered by labia minora and may appear relatively large.

Inspect urethral meatus and vaginal opening

* *Inspect for discharge in infants and children*

EXPECTED: Mucoid whitish discharge is frequently seen during newborn period and sometimes as late as 4 weeks after birth. Discharge may be mixed with blood. UNEXPECTED: Mucoid discharge from irritation by diapers or powder; any discharge in children.

TECHNIQUE	FINDINGS

Assess pubertal development

Assess Tanner stages of female pubic hair development. Six stages of pubic hair development in females.

P_1—Tanner 1 (preadolescent). No growth of pubic hair.

P_2—Tanner 2. Initial, scarcely pigmented straight hair, especially along medial border of the labia.

P_3—Tanner 3. Sparse, dark, visibly pigmented, curly pubic hair on labia.

P_4—Tanner 4. Hair coarse and curly, abundant but less than adult.

P_5—Tanner 5. Lateral spreading; type and triangle spread of adult hair to medial surface of thighs.

P_6—Tanner 6. Further extension laterally, upward, or dispersed (occurs in only 10% of women).

(Growth diagrams from Groningen J, Van Wieringen C, Wafelbakker F, Verbrugge HP, DeHaas JH: Second National Survey on 0-24-Year-Olds, The Netherlands: Noordhoff Uitgevers BV, 1965.)

"Red Flags" for Sexual Abuse

The following signs and symptoms in children or adolescents should raise your suspicion for sexual abuse. Remember, however, that any sign or symptom by itself is of limited significance; it may be related to sexual abuse, or it may be from another cause altogether. This is an area in which good clinical judgment is imperative. Each sign or symptom must be considered in context with the particular child's health status, stage of growth and development, and entire history.

Medical Concerns and Findings

- Evidence of general physical abuse or neglect
- Evidence of trauma and/or scarring in genital, anal, and perianal areas
- Unusual changes in skin color or pigmentation in genital or anal area
- Presence of sexually transmitted infection (oral, anal, genital)
- Anorectal problems such as itching, bleeding, pain, fecal incontinence, poor anal sphincter tone, bowel habit dysfunction
- Genitourinary problems such as rash or sores in genital area, vaginal odor or discharge, pain (including abdominal pain), itching, bleeding, discharge, dysuria, hematuria, urinary tract infections, enuresis

Examples of Nonspecific Behavioral Manifestations

- Problems with school
- Dramatic weight changes or eating disturbances
- Depression
- Anxiety
- Sleep problems or nightmares
- Sudden change in personality or behavior
- Increased aggression and impulsivity or destructiveness
- Sudden avoidance of certain people or places

Examples of Sexual Behaviors That Are Concerning

- Use of sexually provocative mannerisms
- Excessive masturbation or sexual behavior that cannot be redirected
- Age-inappropriate sexual knowledge or experience
- Repeated object insertion into vagina and/or anus
- Child asking to be touched/kissed in genital area
- Sex play between children with 4 or more years of age difference
- Sex play that involves the use of force, threats, or bribes

Modified from Hornor, 2004; Jenny et al, 2013; Kellogg, 2010; Koop, 1988; McClain et al, 2000.

Early Signs of Pregnancy

The following are physical signs that occur early in pregnancy. These signs, along with internal ballottement, palpation of fetal parts, and positive test results for urine or serum human chorionic gonadotropin, are probable indicators of pregnancy. They are considered "probable" because clinical conditions other than pregnancy may cause any one of them. Their occurrence together, however, creates a strong case for the presence of a pregnancy.

SIGN	FINDING	APPROXIMATE WEEKS OF GESTATION
Goodell	Softening of cervix	4 to 6
Hegar	Softening of uterine isthmus	6 to 8
McDonald	Easy flexing of fundus on cervix	7 to 8
Braun von Fernwald	Fullness and softening of fundus near site of implantation	7 to 8
Piskacek	Palpable lateral bulge or soft prominence of one uterine cornu	7 to 8
Chadwick	Bluish color of cervix, vagina, vulva	8 to 12

Sample Documentation

Subjective. A 45-year-old woman has had vaginal discharge and itching for past week. Has had yeast infections before. Completed course of antibiotics for sinusitis 2 days ago. Last menstrual period 2 weeks ago. Sexually active, one partner, mutually monogamous. No unusual vaginal bleeding. Does not douche.

Objective

External: Female hair distribution; no masses, lesions, or swelling. Urethral meatus intact without erythema or discharge. Perineum intact with healed episiotomy scar present. No lesions.

Internal: Vaginal mucosa pink and moist, rugated. No unusual odors. Profuse thick, white, curdy discharge. Cervix pink with horizontal slit midline; no lesions or discharge.

Bimanual: Cervix smooth, firm, mobile. No cervical motion tenderness. Uterus midline, anteverted, firm, smooth, nontender; not enlarged. Ovaries not palpable. No adnexal tenderness or masses.

Rectovaginal: Septum intact. Sphincter tone intact; anal ring smooth and intact. No masses or tenderness.

Male Genitalia

Equipment

- Gloves
- Penlight

EXAMINATION

Have patient lying or standing to start examination.

Spermatic cord

Vas deferens

Pampiniform plexis

Epididymis

Testis

Vas deferens

Vasa efferentia

Testis

Cremasteric muscle

Ductus epididymis

Scrotum

TECHNIQUE	FINDINGS

Wear gloves on both hands

Inspect pubic hair

- *Characteristics*

EXPECTED: Coarser than scalp hair.

- *Distribution*

EXPECTED: Male hair pattern distribution. Abundant in pubic region, continuing around scrotum to anal orifice, possibly continuing in narrowing midline to umbilicus. Penis without hair, scrotum with scant hair.
UNEXPECTED: Alopecia.

Inspect glans penis

- *Uncircumcised patient*
Retract foreskin or ask patient to do so.

EXPECTED: Dorsal vein apparent. Foreskin easily retracted. White, cheesy smegma visible over glans.
UNEXPECTED: Tight foreskin (phimosis). Lesions or discharge.

- *Circumcised patient*

EXPECTED: Dorsal vein apparent. Exposed glans erythematous and dry.
UNEXPECTED: Lesions or discharge.

Examine external meatus of urethra (foreskin retracted in uncircumcised patient)

- *Shape*

EXPECTED: Slitlike opening.
UNEXPECTED: Pinpoint or round opening.

- *Location*

EXPECTED: On ventral surface and only millimeters from tip of glans.
UNEXPECTED: Anyplace other than tip of glans or along shaft of penis.

- *Urethral orifice*
Press glans between thumb and forefinger.

EXPECTED: Opening glistening and pink.
UNEXPECTED: Bright erythema or discharge.

TECHNIQUE	FINDINGS

Palpate penis

Palpate the shaft of the penis.

EXPECTED: Soft (flaccid penis).
UNEXPECTED: Tenderness, induration, or nodularity. Prolonged erection (priapism).

Strip urethra

Firmly compress base of penis with thumb and forefinger; move toward glans.

EXPECTED: No discharge.
UNEXPECTED: Discharge.

Inspect scrotum and ventral surface of penis

- *Color*

EXPECTED: Darker than body skin and often reddened in red-haired patients.

- *Texture*

EXPECTED: Surface possibly coarse. Small lumps on scrotal skin (sebaceous or epidermoid cysts) that sometimes discharge oily material.

- *Shape*

EXPECTED: Asymmetry. Thickness varying with temperature, age, emotional state.
UNEXPECTED: Unusual thickening, often with pitting.

Palpate inguinal canal for direct or indirect hernia

With patient standing, instruct to bear down as if for bowel movement. While patient strains, inspect area of inguinal canal and region of fossa ovalis. Ask patient to relax, and insert examining finger into lower part of scrotum and carry upward along vas deferens into inguinal canal, as shown in figure on p. 190. Ask patient to cough. Repeat examination on opposite side.

EXPECTED: Presence of oval external ring.
UNEXPECTED: Feeling a viscus against examining finger with coughing. If hernia felt, note as indirect (felt within inguinal canal or even into scrotum) or direct (felt medial to external canal).

MALE GENITALIA

MALE GENITALIA

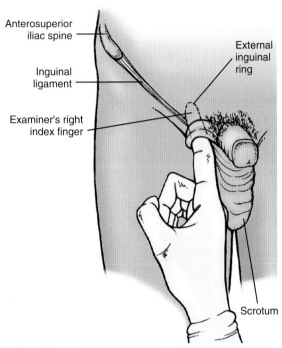

Anterosuperior iliac spine

Inguinal ligament

Examiner's right index finger

External inguinal ring

Scrotum

(From Phipps et al: Medical-Surgical Nursing, ed 8, St. Louis, 2007, Mosby.)

TECHNIQUE	FINDINGS

Palpate testes
Use thumb and first two
fingers. Compress gently.

- *Descent* — EXPECTED: Both testes are present in scrotal sac.
  UNEXPECTED: Cryptorchidism.
- *Consistency* — EXPECTED: Smooth and rubbery. Sensitive to gentle compression.
  UNEXPECTED: Tenderness or nodules. Total insensitivity to painful stimuli.
- *Texture* — UNEXPECTED: Irregular texture.
- *Size* — UNEXPECTED: Irregular size; asymmetry in size, <1 cm or >5 cm.

TECHNIQUE	FINDINGS
Palpate epididymides	
	EXPECTED: Smooth and discrete, with larger part cephalad. UNEXPECTED: Tenderness.
Palpate vas deferens	
Palpate from testicle to inguinal ring. Repeat with other testicle.	EXPECTED: Smooth and discrete. UNEXPECTED: Beaded or lumpy.
Palpate for inguinal lymph nodes	
Ask patient to lie supine, with knee slightly flexed on side of palpation.	EXPECTED: No palpable nodes. UNEXPECTED: Enlarged, tender, red or discolored, fixed, matted, inflamed, or warm nodes and increased vascularity.
Elicit cremasteric reflex bilaterally	
Stroke inner thigh with blunt instrument. Repeat with other thigh.	EXPECTED: The testicle and scrotum rise on the stroked side. UNEXPECTED: Absent reflex.

AIDS TO DIFFERENTIAL DIAGNOSIS

SUBJECTIVE DATA	OBJECTIVE DATA
Hernia	
See table on pp. 192-193.	
Genital Herpes	
Painful lesions on penis; sexually active; may report burning or pain with urination.	Superficial vesicles—located on glans, penile shaft, or base of penis; often associated with inguinal lymphadenopathy.
Condylomata Acuminata (Genital Warts)	
Soft, painless, wartlike lesions on penis. Sexually active.	Single or multiple papular lesions; may be pearly, filiform, fungating (ulcerating and necrotic), cauliflower-like, or plaquelike.
Hydrocele	
Painless enlargement or swelling of the scrotum.	Nontender, smooth, firm mass superior and anterior to the testis. Transilluminates.

SUBJECTIVE DATA	OBJECTIVE DATA
Varicocele	
Usually asymptomatic (and found during evaluation for infertility); may report scrotal pain or heaviness.	Abnormal tortuosity and dilated veins of pampiniform plexus within spermatic cord; described as "bag of worms."
Epididymitis	
Painful scrotum, urethral discharge, fever, pyuria, recent sexual activity.	Possible erythema of overlying scrotum, epididymis feels firm and lumpy, and may be slightly tender, and vasa deferentia may be beaded.
Testicular Torsion	
Acute onset of scrotal pain, often accompanied by nausea and vomiting; absence of systemic symptoms such as fever and myalgia.	Testicle is exquisitely tender; scrotal discoloration often present.
Testicular Cancer	
Painless mass in testicle, scrotal enlargement or swelling; sensation of heaviness in the scrotum, dull ache in the lower abdomen, back, or groin.	Irregular, nontender mass fixed on the testis; does not transilluminate.
Paraphimosis	
Retraction of the foreskin during penile examination, cleaning, urethral catheterization, or cystoscopy; penile pain and swelling.	Glans penis congested and enlarged; foreskin edematous; constricting band of tissue directly behind the head of the penis.

Distinguishing Characteristics of Hernias

	INDIRECT INGUINAL	DIRECT INGUINAL	FEMORAL
Incidence	Most common type of hernia; often patients are children and young males	Less common than indirect inguinal; more common in those older than 40 years	Least common type of hernia; rare in children

	INDIRECT INGUINAL	DIRECT INGUINAL	FEMORAL
Pathway	Through internal inguinal ring; can remain in canal, exit external ring, or pass into scrotum; may be bilateral	Through femoral external inguinal ring; located in region of Hesselbach triangle; rarely enters scrotum	Through femoral ring, femoral canal, fossa ovalis
Presentation	Soft swelling in area of internal ring; pain on straining; hernia comes down canal and touches fingertip on examination	Bulge in area of Hesselbach triangle; usually painless; easily reduced; hernia bulges anteriorly, pushes against side of finger on examination	Right side presentation more common than left; pain may be severe; inguinal canal empty on examination

PEDIATRIC VARIATIONS

EXAMINATION

TECHNIQUE	FINDINGS

Inspect glans penis

- *Uncircumcised patient* Retract foreskin.

EXPECTED: In children, foreskin is fully retractable by age 3 to 4 years. Before that age, forced retraction of foreskin may result in injury. Urethral meatus at tip of penis.
UNEXPECTED: Foreskin adherent in children >4 years. Urethral meatus on dorsal or ventral surface or base of penis.

Palpate scrotum

- *Descent* Palpate testes in children to determine whether testes have descended. If any mass other than testicles or spermatic cord is palpated in scrotum, determine whether it is filled with fluid, gas, or solid material.

EXPECTED: Bilaterally palpable; 1 cm. Considered descended if testis can be pushed into scrotum.
UNEXPECTED: Not palpable unilaterally or bilaterally. If penlight transilluminates, most likely contains fluid (hydrocele). If no light transillumination, most likely a hernia.

MALE GENITALIA

TECHNIQUE	FINDINGS

Evaluate maturation in adolescence

Assess stage of pubertal development

In boys, assess the stage of genital and pubic hair development.

EXPECTED: Tanner stages of male pubic hair and external genital development progress in the sequence shown on pp. 194-195.
UNEXPECTED: Failure to mature and premature maturation.

G_1—Tanner 1. Testes, scrotum, and penis are the same size and shape as in the young child.

G_2—Tanner 2. Enlargement of scrotum and testes. The skin of the scrotum becomes redder, thinner, and wrinkled. Penis no larger or scarcely so.

G_3—Tanner 3. Enlargement of the penis, especially in length; further enlargement of testes; descent of scrotum.

G_4—Tanner 4. Continued enlargement of the penis and sculpturing of the glans; increased pigmentation of scrotum.

G_5 —Tanner 5 (adult stage). Scrotum ample, penis reaching nearly to bottom of scrotum.

Five stages of penis and testes/scrotum development in males. (Growth diagrams from Groningen J, Van Wieringen C, Wafelbakker F, Verbrugge HP, DeHaas JH: Second National Survey on 0-24-Year-Olds, The Netherlands: Noordhoff Uitgevers BV, 1965.)

P₁—Tanner 1 (preadolescent). No growth of pubic hair; that is, hair in pubic area no different from that on the rest of the abdomen.

P₂—Tanner 2. Slightly pigmented, longer, straight hair, often still downy; usually at base of penis, sometimes on scrotum. Stage is difficult to photograph.

P₃—Tanner 3. Dark, definitely pigmented, curly pubic hair around base of penis. Stage 3 can be photographed.

P₄—Tanner 4. Pubic hair definitely adult in type but not in extent (no further than inguinal fold).

P₅—Tanner 5 (adult distribution). Hair spread to medial surface of thighs, but not upward.

P₆—Hair spread along linea alba (occurs in 80% of men).

Six stages of pubic hair development in males. (Growth diagrams from Groningen J, Van Wieringen C, Wafelbakker F, Verbrugge HP, DeHaas JH: Second National Survey on 0-24-Year-Olds, The Netherlands: Noordhoff Uitgevers BV, 1965.)

Sample Documentation

Subjective. A 37-year-old man reports painful burning lesions on his penis. Present past few days. Is sexually active. No burning on urination.

Objective. Hair in male pattern distribution. Circumcised glans without lesions or discharge. Urethral meatus patent on ventral surface at tip of glans. No urethral discharges. Penile shaft with vesicles present. Testes descended bilaterally; smooth without nodularity. Scrotal contents smooth without tenderness. Inguinal areas without bulges or hernias. Inguinal nodes palpable bilaterally. Cremasteric reflex elicited.

17 Anus, Rectum, and Prostate

Equipment

- Gloves
- Water-soluble lubricant
- Light source
- Drapes
- Fecal occult blood testing materials if indicated

EXAMINATION

Have patient in knee–chest or left lateral position with hips and knees flexed, or standing with hips flexed and upper body supported by examining table. *Patients with female genitalia:* Examination usually performed with patient in lithotomy position as part of the pelvic examination. Drape patient appropriately.

TECHNIQUE	FINDINGS
Wear gloves on both hands	
Inspect and palpate sacrococcygeal and perianal area	
• *Skin characteristics*	EXPECTED: Smooth and uninterrupted. UNEXPECTED: Lumps, rashes, tenderness, inflammation, excoriation, pilonidal dimpling, or tufts of hair.

Inspect anus

Spread patient's buttocks. Examine, using penlight or lamp if needed, with patient relaxed, as well as with patient bearing down.

TECHNIQUE	FINDINGS
• *Skin characteristics*	EXPECTED: Skin coarser and darker than on buttocks. UNEXPECTED: Skin lesions, skin tags or warts, external or internal hemorrhoids, fissures and fistulas, rectal prolapse, or polyps.

Inspect, palpate, and assess sphincter tone

Put water-soluble lubricant on index or middle finger; press pad against anal opening, and ask patient to bear down to relax external sphincter. As relaxation occurs, slip tip of finger into anal canal, as shown in the following figure on p. 198. (Assure patient that although he or she may feel the urgency of a bowel movement, it will not occur.) Ask patient to tighten external sphincter around finger.	EXPECTED: Even sphincter tightening. UNEXPECTED: Patient discomfort. Lax or extremely tight sphincter, tenderness.

Palpate muscular anal ring

Rotate finger.	EXPECTED: Smooth, even with consistent pressure exerted. UNEXPECTED: Nodules or other irregularities.

Palpate lateral and posterior rectal walls

Insert finger farther and rotate to palpate lateral, then posterior, rectal walls. If helpful, perform bidigital palpation with thumb and finger by lightly pressing thumb against perianal tissue and bringing finger toward thumb.	EXPECTED: Smooth, even, uninterrupted. UNEXPECTED: Nodules, masses, polyps, tenderness, or irregularities. (Internal hemorrhoids not ordinarily felt unless thrombosed.)

TECHNIQUE   FINDINGS

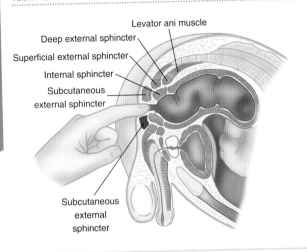

Levator ani muscle
Deep external sphincter
Superficial external sphincter
Internal sphincter
Subcutaneous external sphincter
Subcutaneous external sphincter

Patients with a prostate: Palpate posterior surface of prostate gland through anterior rectal wall

Rotate finger and palpate anterior rectal wall and posterior surface of prostate gland. Alert patient that the feeling of needing to urinate will pass.

- *Consistency and characteristics of anterior rectal wall*

- *Consistency, contour, characteristics of prostate*

EXPECTED: Smooth, even, uninterrupted.
UNEXPECTED: Nodules, masses, polyps, tenderness, or irregularities.
EXPECTED: Surface firm and smooth, lateral lobes symmetric, median sulcus palpable, seminal vesicles not palpable.
UNEXPECTED: Rubberiness, bogginess, fluctuant softness, stony hard nodularity, tenderness, obliterated sulcus, or palpable seminal vesicles.

TECHNIQUE	FINDINGS
• *Size of prostate gland*	EXPECTED: 4-cm diameter with <1 cm protruding into rectum. UNEXPECTED: Protrusion >1 cm (note distance of protrusion). Discharge that appears at urethral meatus (collect specimen for microscopic examination).

Patients with a uterus: Palpate uterus through anterior rectal wall

Attempt to palpate uterus and cervix through anterior rectal wall.

• *Position*	EXPECTED: Midline, retroflexed, or retroverted. UNEXPECTED: Deviation to right or left.
• *Surface characteristics*	EXPECTED: Smooth. UNEXPECTED: Irregular.

Have patient bear down, and palpate deeper

Ask patient to bear down while you reach farther into rectum.	UNEXPECTED: Tenderness of peritoneal area or nodules.

Withdraw finger, and examine fecal material

• *Color and consistency*	EXPECTED: Soft and brown. UNEXPECTED: Blood; pus; or light tan, gray, or tarry black stool. If indicated, fecal material can be tested for blood using a chemical guaiac procedure.

AIDS TO DIFFERENTIAL DIAGNOSIS

SUBJECTIVE DATA	OBJECTIVE DATA

Anal Warts (condyloma acuminata)

Growths on the anus and genitalia.	Single or multiple papular lesions; may be pearly, filiform, fungating (ulcerating and necrotic) cauliflower-like, or plaquelike.

SUBJECTIVE DATA	OBJECTIVE DATA
Perianal and Perirectal Abscesses	
Pain and tenderness in anal area.	Tender, swollen, fluctuant mass; may be draining.
Enterobius Infestation in Children	
Intense perianal itching, especially at night.	Positive tape test. Press the sticky side of cellulose tape against the perianal folds and then press the tape on a glass slide. Nematodes can be seen on microscopic examination.
Anorectal Fissure	
Hard stools; pain, itching, bleeding.	Fissure most often in the posterior midline; spastic internal sphincter.
Anorectal Fistula	
Chills, fever, nausea, vomiting, and malaise.	Elevated, red, granular tissue at external opening, possibly with serosanguineous or purulent drainage on compression of the area; palpable indurated tract.
Hemorrhoids	
Itching and bleeding; discomfort.	May or may not be visible; may be palpable as soft swellings. Thrombosed hemorrhoids appear as blue, shiny masses at anus.
Rectal Carcinoma	
Bleeding; may be asymptomatic.	Sessile polypoid mass with nodular raised edges and areas of ulceration; consistency often stony, with irregular contour.

SUBJECTIVE DATA	OBJECTIVE DATA
Prostatic Carcinoma	
Early carcinoma asymptomatic; symptoms of urinary obstruction as carcinoma advances.	Hard, irregular nodule may be palpable on prostate examination; prostate asymmetric, median sulcus may be obliterated; biopsy required for diagnosis.
Prostatitis	
Acute: Pain, urination problems, sexual dysfunction, fever, chills, shakes. *Chronic:* Asymptomatic, frequent bladder infections, frequent urination, persistent pain in the lower abdomen or back.	*Acute:* Prostate enlarged, acutely tender, and often asymmetric. May have urethral discharge and fever; bacteria in the urine. *Chronic:* Prostate boggy, enlarged, and tender or have palpable areas of fibrosis.
Benign Prostatic Hypertrophy	
Symptoms of urinary obstruction: hesitancy, decreased force and caliber of stream, dribbling, incomplete emptying of the bladder, frequency, urgency, nocturia, and dysuria.	Prostate smooth, rubbery, symmetric, and enlarged; median sulcus may or may not be obliterated.

ANUS, RECTUM, AND PROSTATE

Prostate Enlargement

Prostate enlargement is classified by the amount of protrusion into the rectum:
Grade I: 1 to 2 cm
Grade II: 2 to 3 cm
Grade III: 3 to 4 cm
Grade IV: >4 cm

ANUS, RECTUM, AND PROSTATE

EXAMINATION

TECHNIQUE	FINDINGS
Examine the patency of the anus and its position in all newborn infants. To determine patency, insert a lubricated catheter no more than 1 cm into the rectum.	EXPECTED: Catheter inserts; patency confirmed by passage of meconium. UNEXPECTED: Not able to insert catheter; no evidence of stool.
Inspect perianal area.	UNEXPECTED: Parental concerns about infant's or child's irritability at night or evidence that child has itching in perianal area may indicate presence of parasites such as roundworms or pinworms. Specimen collection and microscopic examination are necessary to confirm findings. Shrunken buttocks suggest a chronic debilitating disease. Asymmetric creases occur with congenital dislocation of the hips. Perirectal redness and irritation are suggestive of pinworms, *Candida,* or other irritants of the diaper area. Rectal prolapse results from constipation, diarrhea, or sometimes severe coughing or straining. Hemorrhoids are rare in children, and their presence suggests a serious underlying problem such as portal hypertension. Small, flat flaps of skin around the rectum (condylomata) may be syphilitic in origin. Sinuses, tufts of hair, and dimpling in the pilonidal area may indicate lower spinal deformities.

Sample Documentation

Subjective. A 57-year-old man is concerned about nighttime urination for the past several months, at least twice per night. Restricts fluid intake after 8 PM. Notices difficulty in starting stream. No pain or bleeding on urination. No change in caliber of stream. Denies change in bowel habits or stool characteristics. No history of prostatitis or enlarged prostate.

Objective. Perianal area intact without lesions or visible hemorrhoids. An external skin tag is visible in the 6 o'clock position. No fissures or fistulas. Sphincter tightens evenly. Prostate is symmetric, smooth, boggy, with 1-cm protrusion into rectum. Median sulcus present. Nontender, no nodules. Rectal walls free of masses. Moderate amount of soft brown stool present.

18 Musculoskeletal System

Equipment

- Goniometer
- Skin-marking pencil
- Reflex hammer
- Tape measure

EXAMINATION

Begin examination as patient enters room, observing gait and posture. During examination, note ease of movement when patient walks, sits, rises, takes off garments, and responds to directions.

TECHNIQUE	FINDINGS

Posture and General Guidelines

Inspect skeleton and extremities, comparing sides

Inspect anterior, posterior, lateral aspects of posture; ability to stand erect; body parts; extremities.

- *Size, alignment, contour, symmetry*
  Measure extremities when lack of symmetry is noted in length or circumference.

EXPECTED: Bilateral symmetry of length, circumference, alignment, position, and number of skinfolds; symmetric body parts; and aligned extremities.
UNEXPECTED: Gross deformity, lordosis, kyphosis, scoliosis, bony enlargement.

Inspect skin and subcutaneous tissues over muscles, cartilage, bones, joints

UNEXPECTED: Discoloration, swelling, or masses.

Inspect muscles and compare sides

- *Size and symmetry*

EXPECTED: Approximately symmetric bilateral muscle size.
UNEXPECTED: Gross hypertrophy or atrophy, fasciculations, or spasms.

MUSCULOSKELETAL SYSTEM

Palpate all bones, joints, surrounding muscles (palpate inflamed joints last)

- *Muscle tone*

EXPECTED: Firm.
UNEXPECTED: Hard or doughy, spasticity.

- *Characteristics*

UNEXPECTED: Heat, tenderness, swelling, fluctuation of a joint, synovial thickening, crepitus, resistance to pressure, or discomfort to pressure on bones and joints.

Test each major joint and related muscle groups for active and passive range of motion, and compare sides

Ask patient to move each joint through range of motion (see instructions for specific joints and muscles in individual sections that follow), then ask patient to relax as you passively move same joints until end of range is felt.

Goniometer.

EXPECTED: Passive range of motion often exceeds active range of motion by 5 degrees. Range of motion with passive and active maneuvers should be equal between contralateral joints.
UNEXPECTED: Pain, limitation of motion, spastic movement, joint instability, deformity, contracture, discrepancies greater than 5 degrees between active and passive range of motion. When increase or limitation in range of motion is found, measure angles of greatest flexion and extension with goniometer, as shown in the following figure, and compare with values as described for specific joints in individual extremities.

Test major muscle groups for strength, and compare contralateral sides

For each muscle group, ask patient to contract a muscle by flexing or extending a joint and to resist as you apply opposing force. Compare bilaterally.

EXPECTED: Bilaterally symmetric strength with full resistance to opposition.
UNEXPECTED: Inability to produce full resistance. Grade muscular strength according to the following table.

Muscle Strength Assessment

MUSCLE FUNCTION LEVEL	GRADE
No evidence of movement	0
Trace of movement	1
Full range of motion, but not against gravity*	2
Full range of motion against gravity but not against resistance	3
Full range of motion against gravity and some resistance, but weak	4
Full range of motion against gravity, full resistance	5

*Passive movement.

TECHNIQUE	FINDINGS

Hands and Wrists

Inspect dorsum and palm of each hand

- *Characteristics and contour*

  EXPECTED: Palmar and phalangeal creases, palmar surfaces with central depression with prominent, rounded mound on thumb side (thenar eminence), and less prominent hypothenar eminence on little-finger side.

- *Position*

  EXPECTED: Fingers able to fully extend and align with forearm when in close approximation to each other.

  UNEXPECTED: Deviation of fingers to ulnar side or inability to fully extend fingers; swan neck or boutonnière deformities.

- *Shape*

  EXPECTED: Lateral finger surfaces gradually tapered from proximal to distal aspects.

  UNEXPECTED: Spindle-shaped fingers, bony overgrowths at phalangeal joints.

TECHNIQUE	FINDINGS

Palpate each joint in hand and wrist

Palpate interphalangeal joints with thumb and index finger, as shown in figure below, panel *A*; metacarpophalangeal joints with both thumbs, as shown in figure below, panel *B*; and wrist and radiocarpal groove with thumbs on dorsal surface and fingers on palmar aspect of wrist, as shown in figure below, panel *C*.

EXPECTED: Joint surfaces smooth.
UNEXPECTED: Nodules, swelling, bogginess, tenderness, or ganglion.

A, Palpating the interphalangeal joints with thumb and index finger. *B*, Palpating metacarpophalangeal joints with both thumbs. *C*, Palpating radiocarpal groove with thumbs on dorsal surface and fingers on palmar aspect of wrist.

Assess integrity of median nerve

- *Tinel sign*
  Strike median nerve where it passes through carpal tunnel with index or middle finger.
- *Thumb abduction test*
  Apply downward pressure on thumb as patient holds thumb perpendicular to hand, palm side up.

UNEXPECTED: Tingling sensation radiating from wrist to hand along pathway of median nerve.
EXPECTED: Full resistance to pressure.
UNEXPECTED: Inability to produce full resistance.

TECHNIQUE	FINDINGS
• *Phalen test* Have patient hold both wrists in fully palmar-flexed position with dorsal surfaces pressed together for 1 minute.	UNEXPECTED: Numbness, paresthesia in distribution of median nerve.
• *Katz hand diagram* Have patient mark specific locations of pain, numbness, tingling in hands and arms on diagram.	UNEXPECTED: Pain, numbness, tingling in pattern shown in the following figure.

Classic pattern
Symptoms affect at least two of digits 1, 2, or 3. The classic pattern permits symptoms in the fourth and fifth digits, wrist pain, and radiation of pain proximal to the wrist, but it does not allow symptoms on the palm or dorsum of the hand.

Probable pattern
Same symptom pattern as classic except palmar symptoms are allowed unless confined solely to the ulnar aspect.
In the **possible pattern,** not shown, symptoms involve only one of digits 1, 2, or 3.

Numbness   Pain   Tingling   Decreased sensation

TECHNIQUE	FINDINGS

Test range of motion

Ask patient to perform the following movements:

- *Metacarpophalangeal flexion and hyperextension*
  Bend fingers forward at metacarpophalangeal joint, then stretch fingers up and back at knuckle.

  EXPECTED: 90-degree metacarpophalangeal flexion and as much as 30-degree hyperextension.

- *Thumb opposition*
  Touch thumb to each fingertip and to base of little finger, then make a fist.

  EXPECTED: Able to perform all movements.

- *Finger abduction and adduction*
  Spread fingers apart and then touch them together.

  EXPECTED: Both movements possible.

- *Wrist extension and hyperextension*
  Bend hand at wrist up and down.

  EXPECTED: 90-degree flexion and 70-degree hyperextension.

- *Radial and ulnar motion*
  With palm side down, turn each hand to right and left.

  EXPECTED: 20-degree radial motion and 55-degree ulnar motion.

Test muscle strength

Ask patient to perform the following movements:

- *Wrist extension and hyperextension*
  Maintain wrist flexion while you apply opposing force.

  EXPECTED: Bilaterally symmetric with full resistance to opposition.
  UNEXPECTED: Inability to produce full resistance.

- *Hand strength*
  Grip two of your fingers tightly.

  EXPECTED: Firm, sustained grip.
  UNEXPECTED: Weakness or pain.

MUSCULOSKELETAL SYSTEM

TECHNIQUE	FINDINGS

Elbows

Inspect elbows in flexed and extended positions

- *Contour*

  UNEXPECTED: Subcutaneous nodules along pressure points of extensor surface of ulna.

- *Carrying angle*
  Inspect with arms at sides passively extended, palms facing forward.

  EXPECTED: Usually 5 to 15 degrees laterally.
  UNEXPECTED: Lateral angle exceeding 15 degrees (cubitus valgus) or a medial carrying angle (cubitus varus).

Palpate extensor surface of ulna, olecranon process, medial and lateral epicondyles of humerus, groove on each side of olecranon process

Palpate with patient's elbow flexed at 70 degrees.

UNEXPECTED: Boggy, soft, tenderness at lateral epicondyle or along grooves of olecranon process and epicondyles.

Test range of motion

Ask patient to perform the following movements:

- *Flexion and extension*
  Bend and straighten elbow.

  EXPECTED: 160-degree flexion from full extension at 0 degrees.

- *Pronation and supination*
  With elbow flexed at right angle, rotate hand from palm side down to palm side up.

  EXPECTED: 90-degree pronation and 90-degree supination.
  UNEXPECTED: Increased pain with pronation and supination of elbow.

Test muscle strength

Ask patient to maintain flexion and extension, as well as pronation and supination, while you apply opposing force.

EXPECTED: Bilaterally symmetric with full resistance to opposition.
UNEXPECTED: Inability to produce full resistance.

TECHNIQUE	FINDINGS

Shoulders

Inspect shoulders, shoulder girdle, clavicles and scapulae, area muscles

- *Size and contour*

EXPECTED: All shoulder structures symmetric in size and contour.
UNEXPECTED: Asymmetry, hollows in rounding contour, or winged scapula.

Palpate sternoclavicular and acromioclavicular joints, clavicle, scapulae, coracoid process, greater trochanter of humerus, biceps groove, area muscles

Palpate the biceps groove by rotating the arm and forearm externally. Follow the biceps muscle and tendon along the anterior aspect of the humerus into the biceps groove.

EXPECTED: No tenderness or masses, bilateral symmetry.

Palpate the muscle insertion for the supraspinatus, infraspinatus, and teres minor near the greater tuberosity of the humerus by lifting the elbow posteriorly to extend the shoulder.

UNEXPECTED: Pain, tenderness, mass.

Test range of motion

Ask patient to perform the following movements:
- *Shoulder shrug*
- *Forward flexion*
  Raise both arms forward and straight up over head.

- *Hyperextension*
  Extend and stretch both arms behind back.

- *Abduction*
  Lift both arms laterally and straight up over head.

EXPECTED: Symmetric rising.
EXPECTED: 180-degree forward flexion.

EXPECTED: 50-degree hyperextension.

EXPECTED: 180-degree abduction.

MUSCULOSKELETAL SYSTEM

TECHNIQUE	FINDINGS
• *Adduction* Swing each arm across front of body.	EXPECTED: 50-degree adduction.
• *Internal rotation* Place both arms behind hips, elbows out.	EXPECTED: 90-degree internal rotation.
• *External rotation* Place both arms behind head, elbows out.	EXPECTED: 90-degree external rotation.

Test shoulder girdle muscle strength

Ask patient to maintain the following positions while you apply opposing force:

• *Shrugged shoulders*
(This also tests cranial nerve XI.)

EXPECTED: Bilaterally symmetric with full resistance to opposition.
UNEXPECTED: Inability to produce full resistance.

Shrugged shoulders.

• *Forward flexion*

EXPECTED: Bilaterally symmetric with full resistance to opposition.
UNEXPECTED: Inability to produce full resistance.

• *Abduction*

EXPECTED: Bilaterally symmetric with full resistance to opposition.
UNEXPECTED: Inability to produce full resistance.

TECHNIQUE	FINDINGS

Assess rotator cuff muscles

Abduct the arm 90 degrees, and flex the shoulders forward 30 degrees to test the supraspinatus muscle. Apply downward pressure on the distal humerus when the arm is rotated so that thumb points down or up.

UNEXPECTED: Pain and weakness with opposing force.

Flex the elbow 90 degrees, and rotate the forearm medially against resistance to test the subscapularis muscle.

UNEXPECTED: Pain and weakness with opposing force.

With the arm at the side and elbow flexed 90 degrees, rotate the arm laterally against resistance to test the infraspinatus and teres minor muscles.

UNEXPECTED: Pain and weakness with opposing force.

Evaluate the rotator cuff for impingement or a tear

- *Neer test:* Have the patient internally rotate and forward flex the arm at the shoulder, pressing the supraspinatus muscle against the anterior inferior acromion.

UNEXPECTED: Increased shoulder pain.

- *Hawkins test:* Abduct the shoulder to 90 degrees, flexing the elbow to 90 degrees, and then internally rotating the arm to its limit.

UNEXPECTED: Increased shoulder pain.

*Assessment for rotator cuff inflammation or tear. **A,** Neer test. **B,** Hawkins test.*

MUSCULOSKELETAL SYSTEM

TECHNIQUE	FINDINGS

Temporomandibular Joint
Palpate joint space for clicking, popping, pain

Locate temporomandibular joints with fingertips placed just anterior to tragus of each ear, as shown in figure at right. Ask patient to open mouth and allow fingertips to slip into joint space. Gently palpate.

EXPECTED: Audible or palpable snapping or clicking may be noted.
UNEXPECTED: Pain, crepitus, locking, or popping.

Palpating temporomandibular joint.

Test range of motion
Ask patient to:
- *Open and close mouth*

- *Move jaw laterally to each side*

- *Protrude and retract jaw*

EXPECTED: Opens 3 to 6 cm between upper and lower teeth.
EXPECTED: Mandible moves 1 to 2 cm in each direction.
EXPECTED: Both protrusion and retraction possible.

Test strength of temporalis and masseter muscles with patient's teeth clenched

Ask patient to clench teeth while you palpate contracted muscles and apply opposing force. (This also tests cranial nerve V motor function.)

EXPECTED: Bilaterally symmetric with full resistance to opposition.
UNEXPECTED: Inability to produce full resistance.

Cervical Spine
Inspect neck from anterior and posterior positions

- *Alignment*

- *Symmetry of skinfolds*

EXPECTED: Cervical spine straight, with head erect and in approximate alignment.
UNEXPECTED: Asymmetric skinfolds, webbed neck.

TECHNIQUE	FINDINGS

Palpate posterior neck, cervical spine, and paravertebral, trapezius, and sternocleidomastoid muscles

EXPECTED: Good muscle tone, symmetry in size.
UNEXPECTED: Palpable tenderness or muscle spasm.

Test range of motion

- *Forward flexion*
  Bend head forward, chin to chest.

  EXPECTED: 45-degree flexion.

- *Hyperextension*
  Bend head backward, chin toward ceiling.

  EXPECTED: 45-degree hyperextension.

- *Lateral bending*
  Bend head to each side, ear to each shoulder.

  EXPECTED: 40-degree lateral bending.

- *Rotation*
  Turn head to each side, chin to shoulder.

  EXPECTED: 70-degree rotation.

Test strength of sternocleidomastoid and trapezius muscles

Ask patient to maintain each of the previous positions while you apply opposing force. (Cranial nerve XI is also tested with rotation.)

EXPECTED: Bilaterally symmetric strength with full resistance to opposition.
UNEXPECTED: Inability to produce full resistance.

Thoracic and Lumbar Spine
Inspect spine for alignment

Note major landmarks of back—each spinal process of vertebrae (C7 and T1 usually most prominent), scapulae, iliac crests, paravertebral muscles.

EXPECTED: Head positioned directly over gluteal cleft, vertebrae straight (as indicated by symmetric shoulder, scapular, and iliac crest heights), curves of cervical and lumbar spines concave, curve of thoracic spine convex, and knees and feet aligned with trunk and pointing directly forward.
UNEXPECTED: Lordosis, kyphosis, scoliosis, or sharp angular deformity (gibbus).

TECHNIQUE	FINDINGS

Palpate spinal processes and paravertebral muscles

Ask patient to stand erect.

UNEXPECTED: Muscle spasm or spinal tenderness.

Percuss for spinal tenderness

Patient is still standing erect. First, tap each spinal process with one finger, then rap each side of spine along paravertebral muscles with ulnar aspect of fist.

UNEXPECTED: Muscle spasm or spinal tenderness.

Test range of motion and curvature

Ask patient to perform the following movements (mark each spinal process with skin pencil if unexpected curvature suspected):

- *Forward flexion*
  Bend forward at waist and try to touch toes. Observe patient from behind to check curvature.

  EXPECTED: 75- to 90-degree flexion; back remains symmetrically flat as concave curve of lumbar spine becomes convex with forward flexion.
  UNEXPECTED: Lateral curvature or rib hump.

- *Hyperextension*
  Bend back at waist as far as possible.

  EXPECTED: 30-degree hyperextension with reversal of lumbar curve.

- *Lateral bending*
  Bend to each side as far as possible.

  EXPECTED: 35-degree lateral bending on each side.

- *Rotation*
  Swing upper trunk from waist in circular motion, front to side to back to side, while you stabilize pelvis.

  EXPECTED: 30-degree rotation forward and backward.

TECHNIQUE	FINDINGS

Test for lumbar nerve root irritation or disk herniation at L4, L5, or S1 levels (patient supine with neck slightly flexed)

- *Straight-leg raising test*
  Ask patient to raise leg with knee extended. Repeat with other leg.

EXPECTED: No pain below knee with leg raising.
UNEXPECTED: Unable to raise leg more than 30 degrees without pain. Pain below knee in dermatome pattern. Flexion of knee often eliminates pain with leg raising. Crossover pain in affected leg.

- *Bragard stretch test*
  Hold patient's lower leg with knee extended, and raise it slowly until pain is felt. Lower leg slightly, briskly dorsiflex foot, and internally rotate hip.

UNEXPECTED: Pain when leg is raised less than 70 degrees; aggravated by dorsiflexion and internal rotation of hip.

Hips

Inspect hips for symmetry and level of gluteal folds

With patient standing, inspect anteriorly and posteriorly, using major landmarks of iliac crest and greater trochanter of femur.

UNEXPECTED: Asymmetry in iliac crest height, size of buttocks, or number and level of gluteal folds.

Test range of motion

While in position indicated, patient should perform the following movements:

- *Flexion, knee extended*
  With patient supine, raise leg over body.

EXPECTED: Up to 90-degree flexion.

- *Hyperextension*
  While standing or prone, swing straightened leg behind body without arching the back.

EXPECTED: Up to 30-degree hyperextension.

MUSCULOSKELETAL SYSTEM

TECHNIQUE	FINDINGS
• *Flexion, knee flexed* While supine, raise one knee to chest while keeping other leg straight.	EXPECTED: 120-degree flexion.
• *Abduction and adduction* While supine, swing leg laterally and medially with knee straight. During adduction movement, lift patient's opposite leg to permit examined leg full movement.	EXPECTED: Some degree of both abduction and adduction.
• *Internal rotation* While supine, flex knee and rotate leg inward toward other leg.	EXPECTED: 40-degree internal rotation.
• *External rotation* While supine, place lateral aspect of foot on knee of other leg. Move flexed leg toward table.	EXPECTED: 45-degree external rotation.

Test hip muscle strength

• *Knee in flexion and extension* Ask patient to maintain flexion of hip with knee in flexion and then extension while applying opposing force.	EXPECTED: Bilaterally symmetric with full resistance to opposition.
• *Resistance to uncrossing legs while seated*	UNEXPECTED: Inability to produce full resistance. EXPECTED: Bilaterally symmetric with full resistance to opposition.

TECHNIQUE	FINDINGS

Perform Trendelenburg test to inspect for weak hip abductor muscles

Ask patient to stand and balance first on one foot, then on other. Observe from behind.

UNEXPECTED: Asymmetry or change in level of iliac crests.

Trendelenburg test. (From Van Tuijl JH, et al: Isolated spinal accessory neuropathy in an adolescent: a case study, Eur J Paediatr Neurol 10(2):83-85, 2006.)

Legs and Knees

Inspect knees and popliteal spaces, flexed and extended

Note major landmarks—tibial tuberosity, medial and lateral tibial condyles, medial and lateral epicondyles of femur, adductor tubercle of femur, patella.

EXPECTED: Natural concavities on anterior aspect, on each side, above patella.
UNEXPECTED: Convex rather than usual concave indentation above patella.

TECHNIQUE	FINDINGS
Observe lower leg alignment	EXPECTED: Angle between femur and tibia less than 15 degrees. Bowlegs common until 18 months of age; knock-knees common between 2 and 4 years. UNEXPECTED: Knock-knees (genu valgum) or bowlegs (genu varum) at other ages, excessive hyperextension of knee with weight bearing (genu recurvatum).
Palpate popliteal space	UNEXPECTED: Swelling or tenderness.
Palpate tibiofemoral joint space Identify patella, suprapatellar pouch, infrapatellar fat pad.	EXPECTED: Smooth and firm joint. UNEXPECTED: Tenderness, bogginess, nodules, or crepitus.
Test range of motion • *Flexion* Ask patient to bend each knee. • *Extension* Ask patient to straighten leg and stretch it.	EXPECTED: 130-degree flexion. EXPECTED: Full extension and up to 15-degree hyperextension.
Test muscle strength • *Flexion and extension* Ask patient to maintain flexion and extension while you apply opposing force.	EXPECTED: Bilaterally symmetric with full resistance to opposition. UNEXPECTED: Inability to produce full resistance.

TECHNIQUE   FINDINGS

Additional Techniques for Knees

Perform ballottement procedure to determine presence of excess fluid or effusion in knee

With knee extended, apply downward pressure on supra-patellar pouch with thumb and finger of one hand, then push patella sharply downward against femur with fingers of other hand, as shown in figure at right. Suddenly release pressure on patella, while keeping fingers lightly on knee.

UNEXPECTED: A tapping or clicking is sensed when patella is pushed against femur. Patella then floats out as if a fluid wave were pushing it.

Ballottement.

Test for bulge sign to determine presence of excess fluid in knee

With knee extended, milk medial aspect of knee upward two or three times, as shown in the following figure, panel *A*, then tap lateral side of patella, as shown in the following figure, panel *B*.

UNEXPECTED: Bulge of returning fluid to hollow area medial to patella.

*Bulge sign. **A,** Milking the medial aspect of the knee two or three times. **B,** Tap the lateral side of the patella.*

TECHNIQUE	FINDINGS

Perform McMurray test to detect torn medial or lateral meniscus

Ask patient to lie supine and flex one knee completely with foot flat on table near buttocks. Maintain that flexion with your thumb and index finger on either side of the joint space while stabilizing knee. Hold heel with other hand; rotate foot and lower leg to lateral position. Extend knee to 90-degree angle. Return knee to full flexion, then repeat procedure rotating foot and lower leg to medial position.

UNEXPECTED: Palpable or audible click or limited extension of knee with either lateral or medial movements.

Procedure for examination of the knee with the McMurray test. Knee is flexed after lower leg was rotated to medial position.

Perform drawer test to identify instability of anterior and posterior cruciate ligaments

Ask patient, while supine, to flex knee 45 to 90 degrees, placing foot flat on table. Place both hands on lower leg with thumbs on ridge of anterior tibia near tibial tuberosity. Pull tibia, sliding it forward of femur. Then push tibia backward.

UNEXPECTED: Anterior or posterior movement greater than 5 mm.

Drawer test.

Perform varus and valgus stress test to identify mediolateral collateral ligament instability

Ask patient to lie supine and extend knee. While you stabilize femur with one hand and hold ankle with other, apply varus force against the ankle (toward midline) and internal rotation.

UNEXPECTED: Excessive laxity felt as joint opening, medial or lateral movement.

TECHNIQUE	FINDINGS

Then apply valgus force against the ankle (away from midline) and external rotation. Repeat with knee flexed to 30 degrees.

Varus and valgus stress test.

Feet and Ankles

Inspect during weight bearing (standing and walking) and non-weight bearing

Note major landmarks—medial malleolus, lateral malleolus, Achilles tendon.

- *Characteristics*

EXPECTED: Smooth and rounded malleolar prominence, prominent heels, prominent metatarsophalangeal joints.
UNEXPECTED: Calluses and corns.

- *Alignment*

EXPECTED: Feet aligned with tibias and weight bearing on foot midline.
UNEXPECTED: In-toeing (pes varus), out-toeing (pes valgus), deviations in forefoot alignment (metatarsus varus or metatarsus valgus), heel pronation, or pain.

- *Contour*

EXPECTED: Longitudinal arch that may flatten with weight bearing. Foot flat when not bearing weight (pes planus) and high instep (pes cavus) are common variations.
UNEXPECTED: Pain with pes planus.

TECHNIQUE	FINDINGS
• *Toes*	EXPECTED: Toes on each foot straight forward, flat, in alignment. UNEXPECTED: Hammertoe; claw toe; mallet toe; hallux valgus; bunions; or heat, redness, swelling, tenderness of metatarsophalangeal joint of great toe (possibly with draining tophus).

Palpate Achilles tendon and each metatarsal joint

Using thumb and fingers of both hands, compress forefoot, palpating each metatarsophalangeal joint.	EXPECTED: No tenderness or masses, bilateral symmetry. UNEXPECTED: Pain, masses, thickened Achilles tendon.

Test range of motion

Ask patient to sit, then perform the following movements:

• *Dorsiflexion* Point foot toward ceiling.	EXPECTED: 20-degree dorsiflexion.
• *Plantar flexion* Point foot toward floor.	EXPECTED: 45-degree plantar flexion.
• *Inversion and eversion* Bend foot at ankle, then turn sole of foot toward and away from other foot.	EXPECTED: 30-degree inversion and 20-degree eversion.
• *Abduction and adduction* Rotate ankle, turning away from and then toward other foot (while you stabilize leg).	EXPECTED: 10-degree abduction and 20-degree adduction.
• *Flexion and extension* Bend and straighten toes.	EXPECTED: Some flexion and extension, especially of great toes.

TECHNIQUE	FINDINGS

Test strength of ankle muscles

Ask patient to maintain dorsiflexion and plantar flexion while you apply opposing force.

EXPECTED: Bilaterally symmetric with full resistance to opposition.
UNEXPECTED: Inability to produce full resistance.

AIDS TO DIFFERENTIAL DIAGNOSIS

SUBJECTIVE DATA	OBJECTIVE DATA

Ankylosing Spondylitis

Develops predominantly in male individuals between 20 and 40 years of age. Begins insidiously with low back pain, also involving hips and shoulders. Pain can fluctuate from one side to the other and progress to reduced spinal mobility.

Restriction in the lumbar flexion of the patient. The shoulders, hips, and knees may be affected later, developing limited range of motion. Uveitis may be present.

Carpal Tunnel Syndrome

Numbness, burning, and tingling in the hands often occur at night. Can also be elicited by rotational movements of the wrist. Pain may radiate to the arms.

Weakness of the hand and flattening of the thenar eminence of the palm may result.

Gout

Sudden onset of a hot, swollen joint; exquisite pain; limited range of motion. Primarily affects men older than 40 years and women of postmenopausal age. Classically affects the proximal phalanx of the great toe, although the wrists, hands, ankles, and knees may be involved.

The skin over the swollen joint may be shiny and red or purple. Uric acid crystals may form as tophi under the skin with chronic gout.

SUBJECTIVE DATA	OBJECTIVE DATA
Lumbar Disk Herniation	
Can be associated with lifting heavy objects. Common symptoms include low back pain with radiation to the buttocks and posterior thigh or down the leg in the distribution of the dermatome of the nerve root. Pain relief is often achieved by lying down.	Spasm and tenderness over the paraspinal musculature may also be present. Patient may have difficulty with heel walking (L4 and L5) or toe walking (S1). Numbness, tingling, or weakness may occur in the involved extremity.
Bursitis	
Common sites include the shoulder, elbow, hip, and knee with pain and stiffness surrounding the joint around the inflamed bursa. The pain usually is worse during activity.	Limitation of motion caused by swelling; pain on movement; point tenderness; and an erythematous, warm site. Soreness may radiate to tendons at the site.
Osteoarthritis	
See table on pp. 227-228.	
Rheumatoid Arthritis	
See table on pp. 227-228.	
Sprain	
Often associated with improper exercise warm-up, fatigue, or previous injury. Severity ranges from a mild intrafibrinous tear to a total rupture of a single muscle.	Temporary muscle weakness, spasm, pain, and contusion.
Fracture	
Usually occurs in the setting of acute trauma. Can occur more easily in patients with bone disorders (e.g., osteogenesis imperfecta, osteoporosis, bone metastasis).	Deformity, edema, pain, loss of function, color changes, and paresthesia.

SUBJECTIVE DATA	OBJECTIVE DATA
Tenosynovitis (tendinitis)	
Pain with movement of such common sites as the shoulder, knee, heel, and wrist.	Point tenderness over the involved tendon. Pain with active movement, and some limitation of movement in the affected joint.
Rotator Cuff Tear	
May be pain in the shoulder and deltoid area that can awaken the patient at night.	May be an inability to maintain a lateral raised arm against resistance. Tenderness over the acromioclavicular joint. Grating sound on movement, crepitus, and weakness in external shoulder rotation.

Differential Diagnosis of Arthritis

SIGNS AND SYMPTOMS	OSTEOARTHRITIS	RHEUMATOID ARTHRITIS
Onset	Insidious	Gradual or sudden (24–48 hours)
Duration of stiffness	Few minutes, localized, but short "gelling" after prolonged rest	Often hours, most pronounced after rest
Pain	On motion, with prolonged activity, relieved by rest	Even at rest, may disturb sleep
Weakness	Usually localized and not severe	Often pronounced, out of proportion with muscle atrophy
Fatigue	Unusual	Often severe, with onset 4 to 5 hours after rising
Emotional depression and lability	Unusual	Common, coincides with fatigue and disease activity, often relieved if in remission
Tenderness over localized afflicted joint	Common	Almost always; most sensitive indicator of inflammation

Continued

MUSCULOSKELETAL SYSTEM

Differential Diagnosis of Arthritis—cont'd

SIGNS AND SYMPTOMS	OSTEOARTHRITIS	RHEUMATOID ARTHRITIS
Swelling	Effusion common, little synovial reaction, swelling rare	Fusiform soft tissue enlargement, effusion common, synovial proliferation and thickening
Heat, erythema	Unusual	Sometimes present
Crepitus, crackling	Coarse to medium on motion	Medium to fine
Joint enlargement	Mild with firm consistency	Moderate to severe

PEDIATRIC VARIATIONS

EXAMINATION

Musculoskeletal findings and motor development in infants, children, and adolescents change as they grow. (For a complete description of age-specific anticipated pediatric findings, see Chapter 21.)

Sports Participation Screening Examination for Children and Adolescents

- Observe posture and general muscle contour bilaterally.
- Observe gait.
- Ask patient to walk on tiptoes and heels.
- Observe patient hop on each foot.
- Ask patient to duck-walk four steps with knees completely bent.
- Inspect spine for curvature and lumbar extension, fingers touching toes with knees straight.
- Palpate shoulder and clavicle for dislocation.
- Check the following for range of motion—neck, shoulder, elbow, forearm, hands, fingers, hips.
- Test knee ligaments for drawer sign.

Sample Documentation

Subjective. A 13-year-old girl referred by school nurse because of uneven shoulder and hip heights. Active in sports, good strength, no back pain or stiffness.

Objective. Spine straight without obvious deformities when erect, but mild right curvature of thoracic spine with forward flexion. Right shoulder and iliac crest slightly higher than left. Muscles and extremities symmetric; muscle strength appropriate and equal bilaterally; active range of motion without pain, locking, clicking, or limitation in all joints.

19 Neurologic System

Equipment

- Penlight
- Familiar objects (coins, keys, paper clip)
- Sterile needles
- Cotton wisp
- Tongue blades (one intact and one broken with pointed and rounded edges)
- Cup of water
- Tuning forks, 200 to 400 Hz and 500 to 1000 Hz
- Reflex hammer
- 5.07 monofilament
- Additional items for a comprehensive diagnostic neurologic examination:
  - Test tubes of hot and cold water
  - Vials of aromatic substances (coffee, orange, peppermint, banana)
  - Vials of solutions (glucose, salt, lemon or vinegar, quinine) with applicators
  - List of tastes

EXAMINATION

Assess the neurologic system as the rest of the body is examined. When history and examination findings have not revealed a potential neurologic problem, perform a neurologic screening examination as shown in the box on p. 231, rather than a full neurologic examination. See Chapter 18 for evaluation of muscle tone and strength, because these findings are important for interpreting neurologic system examination findings. The mental status portion of the neurologic system examination can be found in Chapter 3.

Neurologic Screening Examination

This shorter screening examination is commonly used for health visits when no known neurologic problem is apparent.

Cranial Nerves
Cranial nerves (CNs) II through XII are routinely tested; however, taste and smell are not tested unless some aberration is found (pp. 231-237).

Proprioception and Cerebellar Function
One test is administered for each of the following: rapid rhythmic alternating movements, accuracy of movements, balance (Romberg test), gait, and heel-toe walking (pp. 237-239).

Sensory Function
Superficial pain and touch at a distal point in each extremity are tested; vibration and position senses are assessed by testing the great toe (pp. 240-246).

Deep Tendon Reflexes
All deep tendon reflexes and the plantar reflex are tested, excluding the test for clonus (pp. 247-249).

CRANIAL NERVES I TO XII

The following table summarizes the CN examination, and details of examination follow on pp. 233-237. When a sensory or motor loss is suspected, be compulsive about determining the extent of the loss.

Procedures for Cranial Nerve Examination

CRANIAL NERVE (CN)	PROCEDURE
CN I (olfactory)	Test ability to identify familiar aromatic odors, one naris at a time with eyes closed.
CN II (optic)	Test distance and near vision. Perform an ophthalmoscopic examination. Test visual fields by confrontation and extinction of vision.
CN III, CN IV, CN VI (oculomotor, trochlear, abducens)	Test extraocular movement. Inspect eyelids for drooping. Inspect pupil size for equality, and direct and consensual response to light and accommodation.

Continued

NEUROLOGIC SYSTEM

Procedures for Cranial Nerve Examination—cont'd

CRANIAL NERVE (CN)	PROCEDURE
CN V (trigeminal)	Inspect face for muscle atrophy and tremors. Palpate jaw muscles for tone and strength when patient clenches teeth. Test superficial pain and touch sensation in each nerve branch. (Test temperature sensation if findings to pain and touch sensation are unexpected.) Test corneal reflex.
CN VII (facial)	Inspect symmetry of facial features with various expressions (e.g., smile, frown, puffed cheeks, wrinkled forehead). Test ability to identify sweet, salty, sour, and bitter tastes on each side of tongue.
CN VIII (acoustic)	Test sense of hearing with whisper screening tests or by audiometry. Compare bone and air conduction of sound. Test for lateralization of sound. Test balance with Romberg maneuver.
CN IX (glossopharyngeal)	Test taste sensation (see CN VII). Test gag reflex and ability to swallow.
CN X (vagus)	Inspect palate and uvula for symmetry with speech sounds and gag reflex. Observe for swallowing difficulty. Evaluate quality of guttural speech sounds (presence of nasal or hoarse quality to voice).
CN XI (spinal accessory)	Test trapezius muscle strength (shrug shoulders against resistance). Test sternocleidomastoid muscle strength (turn head to each side against resistance).
CN XII (hypoglossal)	Inspect tongue in mouth and while protruded for symmetry, tremors, atrophy. Inspect tongue movement toward nose and chin. Test tongue strength with index finger when tongue is pressed against cheek. Evaluate quality of lingual speech sounds (l, t, d, n).

TECHNIQUE	FINDINGS

Assess olfactory nerve (CN I)

Ask patient to close eyes. Occlude one naris, hold vial (using least irritating aromatic substances first [e.g., orange or peppermint extract]) under nose, and ask patient to breathe deeply and identify odor. Allow patient to breathe comfortably, then occlude other naris and repeat with different odor. Continue, alternating two or three odors.

EXPECTED: Able to perceive and usually identify odor on each side.
UNEXPECTED: Anosmia, loss of smell or inability to discriminate odors.

Assess optic nerve (CN II)

See tests for near and distance visual acuity and visual fields in Chapter 8.

EXPECTED: Vision 20/20 without or with lenses each eye; full visual fields.

Assess oculomotor, trochlear, abducens nerves (CN III, CN IV, CN VI)

See tests for six cardinal points of gaze, pupil size, shape, response to light and accommodation, and opening of upper eyelids in Chapter 8.

EXPECTED: Equal pupil size, equal and consensual response to light and accommodation, symmetric eye movements in all six cardinal points of gaze.
UNEXPECTED: Absence of lateral gaze. Absence of any expected finding, ptosis.

Assess trigeminal nerve (CN V)

- *Facial muscle tone*
  Inspect face for symmetry or muscle twitching. Ask patient to clench teeth tightly as you palpate muscles over jaw.

EXPECTED: Symmetric tone.
UNEXPECTED: Muscle atrophy, deviation of jaw to one side, or fasciculation.

NEUROLOGIC SYSTEM

TECHNIQUE	FINDINGS

- *Sensation*
  Ask patient to close eyes and report if sensation to touch is sharp or dull as you touch each side of face at scalp, cheek, and chin areas, alternately using sharp and rounded edges of tongue blade or paper clip in an unpredictable pattern. Ask patient to report when the stimulus is felt as you stroke the same six areas with cotton wisp or brush. Finally, test sensation over buccal mucosa with wooden applicator.

EXPECTED: Symmetric discrimination of sensations in each location to all stimuli.
UNEXPECTED: Impaired sensation with identified distribution. If impaired, use test tubes of hot and cold water to evaluate temperature sensation.

Testing sensation over distribution of cranial nerve V.

- *Corneal reflex*
  See test for corneal sensitivity in Chapter 8.

EXPECTED: Symmetric blink reflex. May be diminished or absent if patient wears contact lenses.

Assess facial nerve (CN VII)

- *Expressions*
  Assess motor function by asking patient to make the following facial expressions:
  - *Raise eyebrows and wrinkle forehead*
  - *Smile*
  - *Frown*
  - *Puff out cheeks*
  - *Purse lips and blow out*
  - *Show teeth*
  - *Squeeze eyes shut against resistance*

EXPECTED: Facial symmetry.

Assessing motor function of cranial nerve VII.

NEUROLOGIC SYSTEM

TECHNIQUE	FINDINGS
	UNEXPECTED: Tics, unusual facial movements, or asymmetry of expression (flattened nasolabial fold, lower eyelid sagging, side of mouth drooping).
• *Speech* Listen to articulation and clarity of speech.	UNEXPECTED: Difficulty with enunciation of *b*, *m*, and *p* (labial sounds).
• *Taste (CN VII and CN IX)* Hold card listing tastes in patient's view. Ask patient to extend tongue. Apply one of four solutions to lateral side of tongue in appropriate taste-bud region. Ask patient to point to taste perceived. Offer patient a sip of water, and repeat with different solution and applicator, testing each side of tongue with each solution.	EXPECTED: Able to identify sweet, salty, sour, bitter taste bilaterally when placed in appropriate taste-bud region.

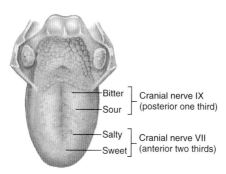

Sites for taste assessment.

TECHNIQUE	FINDINGS

Assess acoustic nerve (CN VIII)

- *Hearing*
  Perform screening tests as described in Chapter 9 or use an audiometer to test hearing.
- *Balance*
  See Romberg test on p. 239.

EXPECTED: Adequate hearing bilaterally.

Assess glossopharyngeal nerve (CN IX)

- *Taste*
  See CN VII.
- *Gag reflex (nasopharyngeal sensation)*
  See CN X.

Assess vagus nerve (CN X)

- *Motor function*
  Ask patient to say "aah" while observing movement of palate and uvula.

  EXPECTED: Soft palate rises with uvula in midline.
  UNEXPECTED: Failure of soft palate to rise or uvula deviates from midline.

- *Gag reflex (nasopharyngeal sensation; CN IX and CN X)*
  Tell patient you will be testing gag reflex. Touch posterior wall of pharynx with applicator while observing palate, pharyngeal muscles, and uvula.

  EXPECTED: Upward movement of palate and contraction of pharyngeal muscles, with uvula in midline.
  UNEXPECTED: Drooping or absence of arch on either side of soft palate; uvula deviates from midline.

- *Swallowing (CN IX and CN X)*
  Ask patient to swallow water.

  EXPECTED: Water easily swallowed.
  UNEXPECTED: Retrograde passage of water through nose.

- *Speech*

  UNEXPECTED: Hoarseness, nasal quality, or difficulty with guttural sounds.

Assess spinal accessory nerve (CN XI)

See Chapters 7 and 18 for evaluations of size, shape, strength of trapezius and sternocleidomastoid muscles of the neck.

EXPECTED: Symmetric size, shape, and strength.

TECHNIQUE	FINDINGS

Assess hypoglossal nerve (CN XII)

- *Tongue resting and protruded*
  Inspect while at rest on floor
  of mouth and while protruded.

Assessing motor function of cranial nerve XII.

EXPECTED: Tongue midline,
symmetric size.
UNEXPECTED: Fasciculation,
asymmetry, atrophy, or deviation from midline.

- *Tongue movement*
  Ask patient to move tongue
  in and out, side to side,
  curled up toward nose, curled
  down toward chin.

EXPECTED: Able to perform
most tongue movements.

- *Tongue strength*
  Ask patient to push tongue
  against cheek while you apply
  resistance with index finger.

EXPECTED: Steady, firm pressure.

- *Speech*

UNEXPECTED: Problems with *l,
t, d,* or *n* (lingual sounds).

Proprioception and Cerebellar Function

Evaluate coordination and fine motor skills

Have patient sit.

- *Rapid, rhythmic, alternating
  movements*
  Ask patient to pat knees with
  both hands, alternately pat-
  ting with palmar and dorsal
  surfaces of the hands. Or
  ask the patient to touch the
  thumb to each finger of the
  same hand sequentially from
  index finger to little finger
  and back, one hand at a time.

EXPECTED: Smooth execution,
maintaining rhythm with
increasing speed.
UNEXPECTED: Stiff, slowed,
nonrhythmic, or jerky clonic
movements.

NEUROLOGIC SYSTEM

TECHNIQUE	FINDINGS
• *Accuracy of movement: Finger-to-nose test* Position your index finger 40-50 cm (15-20 in) from patient. Ask patient to touch his or her nose and your index finger with the index finger of one hand, as shown below. Change location of your index finger several times. Repeat with patient's other hand. Alternatively ask the patient to close both eyes and touch his or her nose with index finger of each hand while alternating hands and gradually increasing speed.	EXPECTED: Movements rapid, smooth, accurate. UNEXPECTED: Consistent past pointing (missing examiner's index finger).

*Assess the patient's accuracy of moving a finger between **A**, the patient's nose, and **B**, the examiner's finger.*

• *Accuracy of movement: Heel-to-shin test (can be performed sitting, standing, or supine).* Ask patient to run heel of one foot along shin of opposite leg from knee to ankle. Repeat with other heel.	EXPECTED: Able to move heel up and down shin in straight line. UNEXPECTED: Irregular deviations to side.

TECHNIQUE   FINDINGS

Evaluate balance

- *Balance: Romberg test*
  Ask patient to stand with feet
  together and arms at sides,
  with eyes first open, then
  closed. **Stand close by in case
  patient starts to fall.**

EXPECTED: Slight swaying
movement, no danger of
falling.
UNEXPECTED: Staggering, losing balance, or swaying to the
extent of falling.

- *Balance: Recovery*
  After explaining test to
  patient, ask patient to spread
  feet slightly, then push shoulders with enough effort to
  throw patient off balance. **Be
  prepared to catch patient.**

EXPECTED: Quick recovery of
balance.
UNEXPECTED: Must catch
patient to prevent a fall.

- *Balance: Standing and hopping*
  Have patient (eyes closed)
  stand in place on one foot,
  then the other. Then have
  patient (with eyes open) hop
  on each foot.

EXPECTED: Able to stand and
hop on each foot for 5 seconds
without losing balance.
UNEXPECTED: Instability, need
to continually touch floor with
opposite foot, or tendency to
fall.

- *Gait: Walking*
  Ask patient to walk without
  shoes around examining
  room or down hallway, with
  eyes open, then closed.

EXPECTED: Smooth, regular
gait, rhythm, and symmetric
stride length; upright trunk
posture swaying with gait
phase; and arm swing smooth
and symmetric.
UNEXPECTED: Shuffling, widely
placed feet, toe walking, foot
flop, leg lag, scissoring, loss of
arm swing, staggering, lurch-
ing, or waddling motion.

- *Gait: Heel-toe walking*
  Ask patient (arms at side and
  eyes open) to walk a straight
  line, first forward and then
  backward. Ask patient to
  touch toes of one foot with
  heel of other.

EXPECTED: Consistent contact
between toe and heel, slight
swaying.
UNEXPECTED: Extension of
arms for balance, instability,
tendency to fall, or lateral
staggering and reeling.

NEUROLOGIC SYSTEM

TECHNIQUE   FINDINGS

Sensory Function

Test primary sensory functions

Ask patient to close eyes for all
tests. Use minimal stimulation
initially, then increase gradually
until patient becomes aware.
Test contralateral areas, asking
patient to compare perceived
sensations side to side.

EXPECTED: For all tests,
minimal differences side to
side, correct interpretation of
sensations (e.g., sharp, dull),
distinguishes side of body
tested and location of sensation (e.g., proximal or distal to
previous stimulus).
UNEXPECTED: For all tests, map
boundaries of any impairment
by distribution of major peripheral nerves or dermatomes
(see figures on pp. 241-242).

TECHNIQUE   FINDINGS

NEUROLOGIC SYSTEM

A

TECHNIQUE   FINDINGS

B

A, Dermatomes of the body, anterior view. *B,* Dermatomes of the body, posterior view.

TECHNIQUE	FINDINGS
• *Superficial touch* Lightly touch skin with cotton wisp or your fingertips, as shown at right. Ask patient to point to area touched or indicate when and where the sensation is felt.	 *Superficial touch assessment.*
• *Superficial pain* Alternate the sharp and smooth edges of broken tongue blade or round and end point of a paper clip, touching the skin in an unpredictable pattern. Allow 2 seconds between sensations. Ask patient to identify sensation (sharp or dull) and where it is felt.	 *Superficial pain assessment.*
• *Temperature and deep pressure* Perform test only if superficial pain sensation is not intact.	
• *Temperature* Alternately roll test tubes of hot and cold water against skin in an unpredictable pattern. Ask patient to indicate hot or cold and where it is felt.	EXPECTED: Distinguishes between hot and cold and location of sensation.
• *Deep pressure* Squeeze trapezius, calf, or biceps muscle.	EXPECTED: Discomfort with deep pressure.

TECHNIQUE	FINDINGS

- *Protective sensation*
Perform test only if patient
has diabetes mellitus or impaired sensation is suspected.
Apply 5.07 monofilament
until filament bends. Use a
random pattern to test several sites on plantar surface
of foot and once on dorsal
surface. Avoid calloused
areas and broken skin.

EXPECTED: Sensation felt at all
sites touched.
UNEXPECTED: Loss of sensation
at any site.

Monofilament testing of superficial touch.

- *Vibration*
Place stem of vibrating
tuning fork against several
bony prominences (e.g., toes,
ankle, shin, finger joints,
wrist, elbow, shoulder,
sternum), beginning distally.
Ask patient when and where
sensation is felt and what
it feels like. Dampen tines
occasionally to see whether
patient notices the difference.

EXPECTED: Buzzing or tingling
sensation, correct location of
stimulus.
UNEXPECTED: Does not distinguish vibration from touch of
nonvibrating tuning fork.

Assessment of vibration sensation.

TECHNIQUE	FINDINGS

- *Position of joints*
  Hold joint to be tested (great toe or finger) by lateral aspects in neutral position, then raise or lower the digit. Ask the patient which way the joint was moved. Return the digit to neutral before moving it another direction. Repeat and test a joint in both feet and both hands.

EXPECTED: Patient correctly identifies position of joint.

Position sense assessment.

Test cortical sensory functions
Ask patient to close eyes for all tests.

- *Stereognosis*
  Hand patient familiar objects (e.g., key, coin) and ask patient to identify by touch.

UNEXPECTED: Inability to recognize objects (tactile agnosia).

Stereognosis.

- *Two-point discrimination*
  Use two paper clip ends or sharp edges of a broken tongue blade, to touch patient's skin with one or both points simultaneously at various locations. Find distance at which patient can no longer distinguish two points.

EXPECTED: Correctly identifies one or two points used. On the fingertips and toes, points are commonly felt when 2 to 8 mm apart. Discrimination of two points varies on other body parts, such as the back (40-70 mm) or chest and forearms (40 mm).

Two-point discrimination.

NEUROLOGIC SYSTEM

TECHNIQUE	FINDINGS

- *Extinction phenomenon*
  Use sharp points of a broken tongue blade to simultaneously touch cheek and hand, or two other areas on each side of body. Ask patient the number of stimuli and locations.

EXPECTED: Correct number and location of both sensations identified bilaterally.

- *Graphesthesia*
  With blunt pen or applicator stick, draw letter, number, or shape on palm of patient's hand, and ask patient to identify it. Repeat with different figure on other hand.

EXPECTED: Letter, number, or figure readily recognized.

Graphesthesia.

- *Point location*
  Touch area on patient's skin and withdraw stimulus. Ask patient to point to area touched.

EXPECTED: Able to locate stimulus.

Reflexes

Test superficial reflexes

Have patient supine.

- *Plantar reflex*
  Using pointed object, stroke lateral side of foot from heel to ball and then across ball of foot to medial side.

EXPECTED: Plantar flexion of all toes. Dorsiflexion of great toe and fanning of other toes in children younger than 2 years.
UNEXPECTED: Fanning of toes or dorsiflexion of great toe with or without fanning of other toes (Babinski sign positive) in all patients older than 2 years.

Plantar reflex assessment.

TECHNIQUE

FINDINGS

- *Abdominal*
  Stroke each quadrant of
  abdomen with end of reflex
  hammer or with tongue
  blade edge.

UNEXPECTED: Slight, bilaterally
equal movements of umbilicus toward each area of stimulation. May have diminished
response in obese patient or
when abdominal muscles
stretched by pregnancy.

Abdominal reflex assessment.

- *Cremasteric (male patients)*
  Stroke inner thigh, proximal
  to distal.

EXPECTED: Testicle and scrotum rise on stroked side.

Test deep tendon reflexes

Patient relaxed and either
sitting or lying for most
procedures. Test each reflex,
comparing responses side to
side. Score deep tendon reflexes
on scale shown in table below.

EXPECTED: Symmetric visible
or palpable responses.
UNEXPECTED: Absent or diminished responses (0 or 1+), or
hyperactive reflexes (3+ or 4+).

Scoring Deep Tendon Reflexes

GRADE	DEEP TENDON REFLEX RESPONSE
0	No response
1+	Sluggish or diminished
2+	Active or expected response
3+	More brisk than expected, slightly hyperactive
4+	Brisk, hyperactive, with intermittent or transient clonus

NEUROLOGIC SYSTEM

TECHNIQUE	FINDINGS

- *Biceps*
Flex arm 45 degrees at elbow, then palpate biceps tendon in antecubital fossa. Place thumb over tendon and fingers under elbow. Strike your thumb with reflex hammer.

EXPECTED: Visible or palpable flexion of elbow, contraction of biceps muscle.

Biceps deep tendon reflex.

- *Brachioradial*
Flex patient's arm up to 45 degrees while resting patient's forearm on your arm, with hand slightly pronated. Strike brachioradial tendon directly.

EXPECTED: Pronation of forearm and flexion of elbow.

Brachioradialis deep tendon reflex.

- *Triceps*
Flex patient's arm at elbow up to 90 degrees. Allow patient's lower arm to hang freely or rest patient's forearm on your arm. Palpate triceps tendon and strike directly with reflex hammer, just above elbow.

EXPECTED: Visible or palpable extension of elbow, contraction of triceps muscle.

Triceps deep tendon reflex.

TECHNIQUE	FINDINGS

- *Patellar*
  Flex patient's knee up to 90 degrees, allowing lower leg to hang loosely. Support upper leg so it does not rest against edge of examining table, then strike patellar tendon just below patella.

EXPECTED: Extension of lower leg, contraction of quadriceps muscle.

Patellar deep tendon reflex.

- *Achilles*
  Ask patient to sit. Then flex patient's knee and dorsiflex ankle up to 90 degrees, holding heel of foot. Strike Achilles tendon at level of ankle malleoli.

EXPECTED: Plantar flexion, contraction of gastrocnemius muscle.

Achilles deep tendon reflex.

- *Clonus*
  Support patient's knee in partially flexed position and briskly dorsiflex foot with other hand, maintaining foot in flexion.

EXPECTED: No rhythmic oscillating movements.
UNEXPECTED: Sustained clonus, rhythmic oscillating movements between dorsiflexion and plantar flexion palpated.

Clonus assessment.

Differential Diagnosis of Upper and Lower Motor Neuron Disorders

ASSESSMENT PARAMETERS	UPPER MOTOR NEURON	LOWER MOTOR NEURON
Muscle tone	Increased tone, muscle spasticity, risk for contractures	Decreased tone, muscle flaccidity
Muscle atrophy	Little or no muscle atrophy, but decreased strength	Loss of muscle strength; muscle atrophy or wasting
Sensation	Sensation loss may affect entire limb	Sensory loss that follows the distribution of dermatomes or peripheral nerves
Reflexes	Hyperactive deep tendon and abdominal reflexes; positive Babinski sign	Weak or absent deep tendon, plantar, and abdominal reflexes, negative plantar reflex, no pathologic reflexes
Fasciculation	No fasciculation	Fasciculation
Motor effect	Paralysis of voluntary movements	Paralysis of muscles
Location of insult	Damage above level of brainstem will affect contralateral side of body, damage below the brainstem will affect the ipsilateral side of the body	Damage affects muscle on ipsilateral side of body

AIDS TO DIFFERENTIAL DIAGNOSIS

SUBJECTIVE DATA	OBJECTIVE DATA

Multiple Sclerosis

Fatigue; vertigo, weakness, numbness; blurred vision, diplopia, vision loss; urinary frequency, urgency, hesitancy; sexual dysfunction; emotional changes	Muscle weakness, ataxia; hyperactive deep tendon reflexes; paresthesias, sensory loss; intention tremor; optic neuritis; cognitive changes

SUBJECTIVE DATA	OBJECTIVE DATA
Generalized Seizure Disorder	
Premonition or aura, stiff body followed by rhythmic jerking movements, eyes rolled upward, drooling; loss of bladder and bowel control	Tonic phase (brief flexion then extension for 10-15 minutes, eyes deviated upward, dilated pupils), clonic phase (alternating muscle contraction and relaxation), postictal (coma followed by confusion and lethargy)
Meningitis	
Fever, chills, headache, stiff neck, lethargy, malaise, vomiting, irritability, seizures	Altered mental status, confusion, nuchal rigidity, may see positive Brudzinski and Kernig signs
Encephalitis	
Recovery from mild viral illness with fever, then onset of lethargy, restlessness, mental confusion	Altered mental status, confusion, stupor, coma, photophobia, stiff neck, muscle weakness, paralysis, ataxia
Intracranial Tumor	
Headaches, may awaken from sleep; nausea and vomiting; memory loss and confusion; unsteady gait, impaired coordination; behavioral or personality changes	Signs vary by location of lesion; altered consciousness, confusion, papilledema, CN impairment, aphasia, vision loss, gait disturbance, ataxia
Stroke (Cerebrovascular Accident [CVA] or Brain Attack)	
Sudden onset of numbness or weakness (often unilateral); sudden confusion, difficulty speaking or understanding speech; sudden trouble seeing in one or both eyes; sudden trouble walking, loss of balance, or loss of coordination; sudden severe headache with no known cause	Altered consciousness, elevated blood pressure, difficulty managing secretions, weakness or paralysis of extremities or facial muscles on one or both sides of body, aphasia (receptive or expressive), articulation impairment, impaired horizontal gaze or hemianopia

NEUROLOGIC SYSTEM

SUBJECTIVE DATA	OBJECTIVE DATA
Parkinson Disease	
Tremors at rest and with fatigue that disappear with intended movement and sleep; slowing of voluntary movement; bilateral pill rolling of fingers; may have numbness, aching, tingling and muscle soreness; difficulty swallowing, drooling	Tremors; muscle rigidity, cogwheel rigidity with jerks; stooped posture; instability of balance; short steps, shuffling, freezing gait; voice softening, slowed, slurred, monotonous speech; impaired cognition, dementia
Peripheral Neuropathy	
Gradual onset of numbness, tingling, burning in hands and feet; sensation of walking on cotton or floors feel strange; inability of fingers to feel difference between coins; night pain in feet	Reduced protective sensation (to pain and touch) in foot and may progress up lower leg; distal pulses diminished, diminished ankle and knee deep tendon reflexes, loss of vibratory sensation below knee, distal muscle weakness, cannot stand on toes or heels
Trigeminal Neuralgia	
Sharp pain episodes on one side of face potentially caused by chewing, swallowing, talking, brushing teeth, or cold exposure	May have slight sensory impairment in regions of pain, may have normal neurologic findings
Bell Palsy	
Rapid progression of muscle weakness on one side of face, feeling of facial numbness	Facial creases and nasolabial fold disappear on affected side, eyelid does not close and lower lid sags on affected side, facial sensation is intact

SUBJECTIVE DATA	OBJECTIVE DATA

Cerebral Palsy

Delays in gross motor development, activity limitation; may have hearing, speech, or language disorders, feeding difficulties

Increased or decreased muscle tone, tremors, scissor gait or wide-based gait, toe walking, exaggerated posturing, cognitive disability or learning disabilities, persistent primitive reflexes, inconsistent muscle tone

PEDIATRIC VARIATIONS

EXAMINATION

Neurologic findings in the infant and child change as the child matures. (For a complete description of expected developmental findings by age, see Chapter 21.)

TECHNIQUE	FINDINGS

Indirectly evaluate CNs in newborns and infants

- *Optical blink reflex (CN II, CN III, CN IV, CN VI)* Shine a light at infant's open eyes. Observe quick closure of eyes and dorsal flexion of head.

EXPECTED: Gazes intensely at close object or face. Focuses on and tracks an object with both eyes.
UNEXPECTED: No response may indicate poor light perception.

- *Rooting reflex (CN V)* Touch one corner of infant's mouth.

EXPECTED: Infant should open mouth and turn head in direction of stimulation. If infant has been fed recently, minimal or no response is expected.

- *Sucking reflex (CN V)* Place your finger in infant's mouth, feeling sucking action. Note pressure, strength, pattern of sucking.

EXPECTED: Tongue should push up against your finger with good strength.

TECHNIQUE	FINDINGS
• *Infant's facial expression (CN VII)* Note wrinkling of forehead when crying and symmetry of smile.	EXPECTED: Facial symmetry with all expressions.
• *Acoustic blink reflex (CN VIII)* Loudly clap your hands about 30 cm from infant's head; avoid producing an air current.	EXPECTED: Blink and movement of eyes in response to sound. Infant will habituate to repeated testing. Freezes position with high-pitched sound. UNEXPECTED: No response after 2 to 3 days of age.
• *Doll's eye maneuver (CN VIII)* Hold infant under axilla in upright position, head held steady, facing you. Rotate infant first in one direction and then in other.	EXPECTED: Infant's eyes turn in direction of rotation and then opposite direction when rotation stops. UNEXPECTED: Eyes do not move in expected direction.
• *Swallowing and gag reflex (CN IX and CN X)* • *Sucking and swallowing (CN XII)* Pinch infant's nose.	EXPECTED: Coordinated sucking and swallowing ability. EXPECTED: Mouth will open, and tip of tongue will rise in midline position.

Evaluate common newborn reflexes in infant

• *Palmar grasp (present at birth)* Making sure infant's head is in midline, touch palm of infant's hand from ulnar side (opposite thumb)	EXPECTED: Strong grasp of your finger. Sucking facilitates grasp. Grasp should be strongest between 1 and 2 months of age and disappear by 3 months.
• *Plantar grasp (present at birth)* Touch plantar surface of infant's feet at the base of toes.	EXPECTED: Toes should curl downward. Reflex should be strong up to 8 months of age.

TECHNIQUE	FINDINGS
• *Moro reflex (present at birth)* With infant supported in semi-sitting position, allow head and trunk to drop back to a 30-degree angle.	EXPECTED: Symmetric abduction and extension of arms. Fingers fan out, and thumb and index finger form a C. Arms then adduct in an embracing motion followed by relaxed flexion. Reflex diminishes in strength by 3 to 4 months and disappears by 6 months.
• *Placing (4 days of age)* Hold infant upright under axilla next to a table or chair. Touch dorsal side of foot to table or chair edge.	EXPECTED: Flexion of hip and knee, lifting of foot as if stepping up on table. Age of disappearance varies.
• *Stepping (between birth and 8 weeks)* Hold infant upright under axilla and allow soles of feet to touch surface of table.	EXPECTED: Alternate flexion and extension of legs, simulating walking. Disappears before voluntary walking.
• *Asymmetric tonic neck or "fencing" (by 2-3 months)* With infant lying supine and relaxed or sleeping, turn infant's head to one side so jaw is over shoulder. Then turn infant's head to other side.	EXPECTED: Extension of arm and leg on side to which head is turned and flexion of opposite arm and leg. Reversal of extremities' positions with head turned opposite way. Reflex diminishes by 3 to 4 months of age and disappears by 6 months. UNEXPECTED: Be concerned if infant never exhibits reflex or seems locked in fencing position.

Sample Documentation

Subjective. A 48-year-old man presents for his annual physical examination. No concerns about poor balance, loss of sensation, unsteady gait. History of diabetes mellitus type 1 for 30 years, reported to be well controlled.

Objective. CNs II to XII grossly intact. Gait is coordinated and even. Romberg negative. Rapid alternating movements coordinated and smooth. Superficial touch, pain, and vibratory sensation are intact bilaterally. Deep tendon reflexes 2+ bilaterally in all extremities. Plantar reflex produces expected plantar flexion of toes. No ankle clonus. Monofilament test reveals decreased sensation on plantar surfaces of both feet.

Head-to-Toe Examination: Adult

Components of the Examination

There are several correct ways to order the physical examination. You are encouraged to consider and then to adapt the following suggested approach for the unique needs of the particular patient and the relevant demands of the moment.

GENERAL INSPECTION

Start the examination the moment the patient is within your view. As you first observe the patient, for example, in the waiting room, take note of the following characteristics:

- Signs of distress or disease
- Habitus
- Manner of sitting
- Degree of facial relaxation

- Relationship with others in room
- Degree of interest in what is happening in room

- Manner with which you are met
- Moistness of palm when you shake hands
- Facial expression
- Eyes—luster and expression of emotion
- Eye contact with you
- Skin color
- Mobility:
  - Use of assistive devices
  - Gait
  - Sitting, rising from chair
  - Taking off coat
- Stature, build
- Musculoskeletal deformities
- Dress, posture
- Speech pattern, disorders, foreign language
- Difficulty hearing, assistive devices
- Vision problems, assistive devices
- Orientation, mental alertness
- Nutritional state
- Respiratory problems
- Significant others accompanying patient

PATIENT INSTRUCTIONS (PLAN EACH STEP TO MINIMIZE THE PATIENT'S EFFORT AND TO CONSERVE ENERGY)

- Empty bladder.
- Remove as much clothing as is necessary (always respecting modesty).
- Put on a gown.

MEASUREMENTS

- Measure weight and height.
- Calculate the body mass index.
- Assess distance vision—Snellen chart.
- Document vital signs—temperature, pulse, respiration, blood pressure in both arms, pain assessment.

PATIENT SEATED, WEARING GOWN

Stand in front of patient seated on examining table.

Head and Face

- Inspect skin characteristics.
- Inspect symmetry and external characteristics of eyes and ears.
- Inspect configuration of skull.
- Inspect and palpate scalp and hair for texture, distribution, and quantity of hair.
- Palpate facial bones.
- Palpate temporomandibular joint while patient opens and closes mouth.
- Palpate sinus regions; if tender, transilluminate them (may be helpful, but sensitivity and specificity are uncertain when considered separate from other findings).
- Inspect ability to clench teeth, squeeze eyes tightly shut, wrinkle forehead, smile, stick out tongue, and puff out cheeks (cranial nerve [CN] V, VII).
- Test sensation using light touch on forehead, cheeks, chin (CN V).

Eyes

- External examination:
    - Inspect eyelids, eyelashes, palpebral folds.
    - Determine alignment of eyebrows.
    - Inspect sclerae, conjunctivae, irides.
    - Palpate lacrimal apparatus.
    - Test near-vision—Rosenbaum chart (CN II).
- Eye function:
    - Test pupillary response to light and accommodation.
    - Perform cover–uncover test and corneal light reflex.

- Test extraocular eye movements (CN III, IV, VI).
- Assess visual fields (CN II).
- Test corneal reflexes (CN V).
- Ophthalmoscopic examination:
  - Test red reflex.
  - Inspect lens.
  - Inspect disc, cup margins, vessels, retinal surface.

Ears

- Inspect alignment and placement.
- Inspect surface characteristics.
- Palpate auricle.
- Assess hearing with whisper test or ticking watch (CN VIII).
- Perform otoscopic examination:
  - Inspect canals.
  - Inspect tympanic membranes for landmarks, deformities, inflammation.
- Perform Rinne and Weber tests.

Nose

- Note structure, position of septum.
- Determine patency of each nostril.
- Inspect mucosa, septum, turbinates with nasal speculum.
- Assess sense of smell when clinically necessary (CN I).

Mouth and Pharynx

- Inspect lips, buccal mucosa, gums, hard and soft palates, floor of mouth for color and surface characteristics.
- Inspect oropharynx: Note anteroposterior pillars, uvula, tonsils, posterior pharynx, mouth odor.
- Inspect teeth for color, number, surface characteristics.
- Inspect tongue for color, characteristics, symmetry, movement (CN XII).
- Test gag reflex and "aah" reflex (CN IX, X).
- Test sense of taste when clinically indicated (CN VII, IX).

Neck

- Inspect for symmetry and smoothness of neck and thyroid.
- Inspect for jugular venous distention (also when patient is supine).
- Perform active and passive range of motion; test resistance against examiner's hand.

- Test strength of shoulder shrug (CN IX).
- Palpate carotid pulses. Be sure to palpate one side at a time (also when patient is supine).
- Palpate tracheal position.
- Palpate thyroid.
- Palpate lymph nodes—preauricular and postauricular, occipital, tonsillar, submental, submandibular, superficial cervical chain, posterior cervical, deep cervical, supraclavicular.
- Auscultate carotid arteries and thyroid.

Upper Extremities

- Inspect skin and nail characteristics.
- Inspect symmetry of muscle mass.
- Inspect and palpate hands, arms, shoulders, including epitrochlear nodes; note musculoskeletal deformities.
- Assess joint range-of-motion and muscle strength: fingers, wrists, elbows, and shoulders.
- Assess pulses—radial, brachial.

PATIENT SEATED, BACK EXPOSED

Stand behind patient seated on examining table. Have male patients pull gown down to the waist so entire chest and back are exposed. Have females expose back; keep breasts covered.

Back and Posterior Chest

- Inspect skin and thoracic configuration.
- Inspect symmetry of shoulders, musculoskeletal development.

- Inspect and palpate scapulae and spine.
- Palpate and percuss costovertebral angle.

Lungs

- Inspect chest movement with respiration—excursion, depth, rhythm, pattern.
- Palpate for expansion and tactile fremitus.
- Palpate scapular and subscapular nodes.
- Percuss posterior chest and lateral walls systematically for resonance.
- Percuss for diaphragmatic excursion.
- Auscultate systematically for breath sounds. Note characteristics and adventitious sounds.

PATIENT SEATED, CHEST EXPOSED

Move around to front of patient. Have female patients lower gown to expose anterior chest.

Anterior Chest, Lungs, Heart

- Inspect skin, musculoskeletal development, symmetry.
- Inspect chest movement with respirations—patient posture, respiratory effort.
- Inspect for pulsations or heaving.
- Palpate chest wall for stability, crepitation, tenderness.
- Palpate precordium for thrills, heaves, pulsations, and location of apical impulse.

- Palpate for tactile fremitus.
- Palpate axillary nodes.
- Percuss systematically for resonance.
- Auscultate systematically for breath sounds.
- Auscultate systematically for heart sounds—aortic, pulmonic, second pulmonic, tricuspid, and mitral areas.

Female Breasts

- Inspect in these positions—patient's arms hanging loosely at the sides, extended over head or flexed behind the neck, pushing hands on hips, hands pushed together in front of chest, patient leaning forward.
- Perform chest wall sweep from clavicles to nipples.
- Perform bimanual digital palpation of each breast.
- Palpate for axillary, supraclavicular, and infraclavicular lymph nodes (if not already performed).

Male Breasts

- Inspect breasts and nipples for symmetry, enlargement, surface characteristics.
- Palpate breast tissue.
- Palpate for axillary, supraclavicular, and infraclavicular lymph nodes.

PATIENT RECLINING 45 DEGREES

- Assist patient to a reclining position at a 45-degree angle. Stand to side of patient that allows greatest comfort and approach for examination.
- Inspect chest in recumbent position.
- Inspect jugular venous pulsations; measure right jugular venous pressure.

PATIENT SUPINE, CHEST EXPOSED

Assist patient into supine position. If patient cannot tolerate lying flat, maintain head elevation at 30-degree angle. Uncover chest while keeping abdomen and lower extremities draped.

Female Breasts

- Inspect and palpate with patient in recumbent position with patient's arm over the head on same side being examined. Use light, medium, and deep palpation of breast.
- Depress nipple into well behind the areola.

Heart

- Palpate chest wall for thrills, heaves, pulsations.
- Auscultate systematically; turn patient slightly to left side and repeat auscultation.

PATIENT SUPINE, ABDOMEN EXPOSED

Have patient remain supine. Cover chest with patient's gown. Arrange draping to expose abdomen from pubis to epigastrium.

Abdomen

- Inspect skin characteristics, contour, pulsations, movement.
- Auscultate all quadrants for bowel sounds.
- Auscultate aorta and renal, iliac, and femoral arteries for bruits or venous hums.
- Percuss all quadrants for tone.
- Percuss liver borders and estimate span.
- Percuss left midaxillary line for splenic dullness.
- Lightly palpate all quadrants.
- Deeply palpate all quadrants.
  - Palpate right costal margin for liver border.
  - Palpate left costal margin for spleen.

- Palpate at the flanks for right and left kidneys.
- Palpate midline for aortic pulsation.
- Test abdominal reflexes.
- Have patient raise head as you inspect abdominal muscles.

Inguinal Area

- Palpate for lymph nodes, pulses, hernias.

External Genitalia, Males

- Inspect penis, urethral meatus, scrotum, pubic hair.
- Palpate scrotal contents.
- Test cremasteric reflex.

PATIENT SUPINE, LEGS EXPOSED

Have patient remain supine. Arrange drapes to cover abdomen and pubis, and to expose lower extremities.

Feet and Legs

- Inspect for skin characteristics, hair distribution, muscle mass, musculoskeletal configuration.
- Palpate for temperature, texture, edema, pulses (dorsalis pedis, posterior tibial, popliteal).
- Test range of motion and strength of toes, feet, ankles, knees.

Hips

- Palpate hips for stability.
- Test range of motion and strength of hips.

PATIENT SITTING, LAP DRAPED

Assist patient to a sitting position. Have patient wear gown with a drape across lap.

Musculoskeletal

- Observe patient moving from lying to sitting position.
- Note coordination, use of muscles, ease of movement.

Neurologic

- Test sensory function—dull and sharp sensation of forehead, cheeks, chin, lower arms, hands, lower legs, feet.
- Test position sense and vibratory sensation of wrists, ankles.
- Test two-point discrimination of palms, thighs, back.
- Test stereognosis, graphesthesia.
- Test fine motor function, coordination, and position sense of upper extremities, asking patient to do the following:
  - Touch nose with alternating index fingers.
  - Rapidly alternate touching fingers to thumb.
  - Rapidly move index finger between own nose and examiner's finger.
- Test fine motor function, coordination, and position sense of lower extremities, asking patient to do following:
  - Run heel down tibia of opposite leg.
- Test deep tendon reflexes and compare bilaterally—biceps, triceps, brachioradial, patellar, Achilles.
- Test plantar reflex bilaterally.

PATIENT STANDING

Assist patient to standing position. Stand next to patient.

Spine

- Inspect and palpate spine as patient bends over at waist.
- Test range of motion—hyperextension, lateral bending, rotation of upper trunk.

Neurologic

- Observe gait.
- Test proprioception and cerebellar function:
  - Perform Romberg test.
  - Ask patient to walk heel to toe.
  - Ask patient to stand on one foot, then the other, with eyes closed.
  - Ask patient to hop in place on one foot, then other, with eyes open.

Abdominal/Genital

- Test for inguinal and femoral hernias.

FEMALE PATIENT, LITHOTOMY POSITION

Assist female patient into lithotomy position and drape appropriately. Examiner is seated.

External Genitalia

- Inspect pubic hair, labia, clitoris, urethral opening, vaginal opening, perineal and perianal area, anus.
- Palpate labia and Bartholin glands; milk Skene glands.

Internal Genitalia

- Perform speculum examination:
  - Inspect vagina and cervix.
  - Collect Pap smear/human papillomavirus and other necessary specimens.
- Perform bimanual palpation to assess for characteristics of vagina, cervix, uterus, adnexa (examiner standing).
- Perform rectovaginal examination to assess rectovaginal septum, broad ligaments.
- Perform rectal examination:
  - Assess anal sphincter tone and surface characteristics; palpate circumferentially for rectal mass.
  - Obtain rectal culture if needed.
  - Note characteristics of stool when gloved finger is removed. Test for occult blood.

MALE PATIENT, BENDING FORWARD

- Assist male patient in leaning over examining table (or into knee-chest or lateral decubitus position). Stand behind patient.
- Inspect sacrococcygeal and perianal areas.
- Perform rectal examination:
  - Palpate sphincter tone and surface characteristics.
  - Obtain rectal culture if needed.

- Palpate prostate gland and seminal vesicles.
- Note characteristics of stool when gloved finger is removed. Test for occult blood.

CONCLUSION

- Allow patient to dress in private.
- Share findings and interpretations with patient.
- Answer the patient's additional questions.
- Confirm that the patient has a clear understanding of all aspects of the situation.
- If patient is examined in a hospital bed:
  - Put everything back in order when finished.
  - Make sure patient is comfortably settled in an appropriate manner.
  - Put bed side rails up if clinical condition warrants it.
  - Make sure buttons and buzzers are within easy reach.

21 Age-Specific Examination: Infants, Children, and Adolescents

Examination Guidelines

A pediatric physical examination must, of course, be age and developmentally appropriate. Not every observation and examination maneuver must be made on every child at every examination. What you do depends on the individual circumstance and your clinical judgment, each step dependent on the patient's age, physical condition, and emotional state. The order of the examination can and should be modified according to need. There is no one right way. The safety of the child on the examining table must be ensured. During most of infancy and into the pre-elementary school years (and even later), an adult's lap is most often a more secure surface for much and often all of the examination.

- In the medical record, describe child's behavior and nature of the relationship during interactions with parent (or caregiver) and with you.
- Offer toys, a book, or paper and crayons to entertain child (if age appropriate), to develop rapport, and to assist you in assessing child's development and neurologic status. Attempt to gain child's cooperation and build rapport, even if it takes more time; future visits will be more pleasant for both of you.
- Only if absolutely necessary, restrain child for funduscopic, otoscopic, oral examinations; restraint is easier on an adult lap with the aid of the adult.
- Lessen fear of these examinations by permitting child to handle instruments, blow out light, or use them on a doll, a parent, or yourself.
- Record temperature, weight, length, or height; also take blood pressure (record extremity or extremities used, size of cuff, and method used).
- Note percentiles for all measurements, including body mass index for children 2 years and older.

- If clinical issues require it, include arm span, upper segment measurement (crown to top of symphysis), lower segment measurement (symphysis to soles of feet), upper/lower segment ratio, and chest circumference.
- Review parent-completed developmental screening tool to assess language, motor abilities, social skills, and parental concerns.
- Evaluate mental status as child interacts with you and parent.

CHILD PLAYING

- While child plays, evaluate musculoskeletal and neurologic system while developing rapport with child.
- Observe child's spontaneous activities.
- Ask child to demonstrate skills: turning pages in a book, building block towers, drawing geometric figures, coloring.
- Evaluate gait, jumping, hopping, range of motion.
- Observe child climbing on parent's lap, stooping, and recovering.

CHILD ON PARENT'S LAP

- Perform examination on parent's lap; the adult and the patient generally enjoy the experience more, and you, sitting on a stool, preferably with your eyes at the child's eye level, will find it easier than the examining table.
- Begin with child sitting and undressed except for diaper or underpants.

Upper Extremities

- Inspect arms for movement, size, shape, and skin lesions; observe use of hands; inspect hands for number and configuration of fingers, palmar creases.
- Palpate radial pulses.
- Elicit biceps and triceps reflexes.
- Check blood pressure if not previously taken.

Lower Extremities

- Child may stand for much or part of examination.
- Inspect legs for movement, size, shape, alignment, lesions.
- Inspect feet for alignment, longitudinal arch, number of toes.
- Palpate femoral and dorsalis pedis pulses.
- Elicit plantar, Achilles, and patellar reflexes.

Head and Neck

- Inspect head.
- Inspect shape, alignment with neck, hairline, eyelids, palpebral folds, conjunctivae, sclerae, irides, position of auricles.
- Palpate anterior fontanel for size (age appropriate); head for sutures, depressions; hair for texture.
- Measure head circumference (up to age 36 months).
- Inspect neck for webbing, voluntary movement.
- Palpate neck: thyroid, muscle tone, lymph nodes, position of trachea.

Chest, Heart, Lungs

- Inspect chest for respiratory movement, size, shape, precordial movement, deformity, nipple and breast development.
- Palpate anterior chest, locate point of maximal impulse.
- Auscultate anterior, lateral, and posterior chest for breath sounds; count respirations.
- Auscultate all cardiac listening areas for S_1 and S_2, splitting, murmurs; count apical pulse.

CHILD RELATIVELY SUPINE, STILL ON LAP, DIAPER LOOSENED

- Inspect abdomen.
- Auscultate for bowel sounds.
- Palpate: Identify size of liver and any other palpable organs or masses.
- Percuss.
- Palpate femoral pulses; compare with radial pulses.
- Palpate for inguinal lymph nodes.
- Inspect external genitalia.
- Males: Palpate scrotum for descent of testes and other masses.

CHILD STANDING

- Inspect spinal alignment as child bends slowly forward to touch toes.
- Observe posture from anterior, posterior, lateral views.
- Observe gait.

CHILD ON PARENT'S LAP

The following steps, often delayed to the end of the examination, are more easily performed with a child of appropriate age sitting on a parent's or caregiver's lap.

- Inspect eyes: pupillary light reflex, red reflex, corneal light reflex, extraocular movements, funduscopic examination.
- Perform otoscopic examination. Note position and description of pinnae.
- Inspect nasal mucosa.
- Inspect mouth and pharynx. Note number of teeth, deciduous or permanent, and any special characteristics.

NOTE: By the time child is of school age, it is usually possible to use an examination sequence very similar to that for adults.

Age-Specific Anticipated Observations and Guidelines

Again, this is a suggested outline, always modified by human variation, and all percentages are subject to Gaussian distribution. History building can be facilitated by referring to baby books, report cards, photos on mobile devices, and other materials the family may have at home.

BIRTH TO 2 WEEKS OF AGE

History (particular attention)
- Pertinent perinatal and maternal history
- Social: caregiver arrangements, housing
- Maternal mood and social support
- Stool pattern
- Umbilicus: healing, discharge, granulation
- Diet: feeding modality, schedule
- Sleep environment

Development

By this age:

- 80% will lift and turn head when in prone position.
- 40% will follow an object to midline visually.
- 35% will vocalize, become quiet in response to a voice.
- 45% will regard a face intently, diminishing activity for the moment.

Physical Examination (particular attention)

- Establish growth curves (weight, height, head circumference).
- Examine hips.
- Test reflexes: Moro, root, grasp, step.

Anticipatory Guidance (particular attention)

- Sleep: emphasize supine position and safe sleep environment (alone, back, crib or bassinet)
- Feeding: use of pacifier (need to suck)
- Use of bulb syringe (nasal stuffiness)
- Safety: falling, crib, car seats, hot water temperature for bathing
- Skin care
- Clothing
- Illness: temperature taking
- Crying (holding the baby)

Plans and Problems

- What risks have revealed themselves as you have gotten to know the family? What are apparent problems? Start a problem list and make appropriate recommendations.
- Review results of newborn metabolic screening, hearing screening, and any other notable medical issues requiring follow-up.
- Consider immunization needs and, throughout, attempt to follow American Academy of Pediatrics guidelines; on each visit, discuss benefits, risks, and side effects of immunizations (always remember risks for the immunocompromised).

2 MONTHS OF AGE

History (particular attention)

- Expressions of parental concern
- Child's apparent temperament
- Sleep cycle

- Safe sleep positioning and environment
- Feeding patterns, frequency
- Stooling pattern, frequency, color, consistency, straining
- Social issues:
  Maternal mood
  Father's involvement
  Living conditions
  Smoking, other concerning environmental exposures
  Any apparent high-risk concerns

Development

By this age:
- Gross motor:
  80% will lift head to 45 degrees in prone position.
  45% will lift head to as much as 90 degrees in prone position.
  25% will roll over from stomach to back.
- Fine motor:
  ≥99% will follow a moving object to midline.
  85% will follow a moving object past midline.
- Language:
  Almost all will diminish activity at the sound of a voice.
  35% will spontaneously vocalize.
  Many will vocalize responsively.
- Psychosocial:
  Almost all will diminish activity when regarding a face.
  Almost all will respond to a friendly, cooing face with a social smile.
  50% may smile spontaneously or even laugh aloud.

Physical Examination (particular attention)

- Growth curves (weight, height, head circumference)
- Hearing
- Vision
- Hips

Anticipatory Guidance

- Feeding
- Childcare arrangements when and if mother returns to work
- Hiccups
- Straining at stool

- Visual and auditory stimulus (mobiles, mirrors, rattles, singing and talking to baby)
- Sibling rivalry (if there are siblings or other children in home)
- Babysitters and other caregivers (checking references, reliability)
- Safety (rolling over, playpen, car seat, smoke detectors in home)
- Sleep (reemphasize location and supine position)
- Smoking in home and contribution to poor health

Plans and Problems

- Review immunizations, and provide as appropriate.
- List problems (e.g., allergies, medications, any areas of concern), and make appropriate plans and, if necessary, referrals.

4 MONTHS OF AGE

History (particular attention)

- Parental concerns
- Infant's sleep cycle
- Safe sleep positioning and environment
- Temperament
- Feeding patterns, frequency
- Stooling pattern, frequency, color, consistency, straining
- Social issues:
  Maternal mood
  Father's involvement
  Review family structure and social supports
  Smoking, other concerning environmental exposures
  Any apparent high-risk concerns

Development

By this age:

- Gross motor:
  80%, when prone, will lift chest up with arm support.
  80% will roll over from stomach to back.
  35% will have no head lag when pulled to sitting position, and many will then hold head steady when kept in that position.
- Fine motor:
  60% will reach for a dangling object.
  Almost all will bring hands together.
  Almost all will follow a face or object up to 180 degrees.
- Language:
  Almost all will laugh aloud.
  20% will appear to initiate vocalization.

- Psychosocial:
  80% will smile spontaneously.
  Many will regard their own hand for several seconds.

Physical Examination (particular attention)

- Update growth curves (weight, height, head circumference).
- Reassess hearing.
- Reassess vision.

Anticipatory Guidance

- Introduction of solid food (iron-fortified cereal)
- Stool changes with changes in diet
- Drooling and teething
- Thumb sucking, pacifiers, bottles at bedtime
- Safety (aspiration, rolling over, holding baby with hot liquids, reemphasize earlier discussions [e.g., car seat])
- Reemphasis on environmental stimulus
- Further discussion of babysitters and other caregivers
- Use of antipyretics (e.g., acetaminophen)

Plans and Problems

- Review immunizations, and provide as appropriate.
- Maintain problem list, making appropriate plans and, if necessary, referrals.

6 MONTHS OF AGE

History (interim details)

- Parental concerns
- Sleep patterns
- Diet
- Stooling pattern
- Further exploration of social issues
- If either parent has not attended these care visits regularly, encourage his or her participation and address relevant issues.

Development

By this age:

- Gross motor:
  90%, pulled to a sitting position, will have no head lag.
  60% will sit alone.
  75% will bear some weight on legs.
  Almost all will roll over.

- Fine motor:
  More than half will pass a toy from hand to hand.
  60%, in a sitting position, will look for a toy.
  40%, in a sitting position, will take two cubes.
- Language:
  60% will turn toward a voice.
  30% will initiate speech sounds (e.g., "mama," "dada") but not specifically.
- Psychosocial:
  30% may cry and turn away from strangers.
  40% may put an object in mouth to explore it, may feed self.
  60% may resist an attempt to pull away an object while holding it.

Physical Examination (particular attention)

- Update growth curves.
- Double-check hearing and vision.
- Look for any new findings, and recheck prior findings.

Anticipatory Guidance

- Bedtime routines (discuss putting child to bed while child is awake; waking up at night)
- Fear of strangers
- Separation anxiety
- Safety (begin discussions about what toddlers can get into, cabinets, hot water, electrical outlets, medications and other poisons; inform about local poison control center)
- Shoes, when and if to use them
- Teething, oral hygiene
- Offering a cup
- Checking fluoride intake
- Addition of solid foods

Plans and Problems

- Review immunizations, and provide as appropriate.
- Maintain problem list, making appropriate plans and, if necessary, referrals.

9 MONTHS OF AGE

History (interim details)

- Parental concerns
- Continued attention to sleep, diet, stooling patterns
- Continued attention to social issues

Development

By this age:

- Gross motor:
  Almost 100% will sit alone.
  80% will stand alone.
  45% will cruise.
  Some will have begun competent crawling.
- Fine motor:
  70% will have thumb-finger grasp.
  60% will bang two cubes together.
  Almost all will finger feed.
- Language:
  75% will imitate speech sounds.
  75% will use "mama," "dada" nonspecifically.
- Psychosocial:
  Almost 100% will try to get to a toy that is out of reach.
  85% will play repetitive games (e.g., peekaboo).
  45% will be shy with strangers and may cry.

Physical examination (particular attention)

- Update growth curves.
- Reassess earlier findings, and note any new findings.

Anticipatory guidance

- Oral hygiene—for example, water without sugar in bottles (avoid tooth decay)
- Sleep and desirability of routine (naps, separation anxiety, and how to deal with it)
- Reemphasis on checking references and reliability of babysitters and caregivers
- Safety—for example, stair gates and toddlers, falls, poisoning, burns, aspiration (never enough emphasis on safety, smoking in the home, etc.)
- Weaning, breast and/or bottle
- Uses of discipline

Plans and Problems

- Review immunizations, and provide as appropriate.
- Perform developmental screening (using parent-administered validated tool).
- Consider need for a serum lead level, hemoglobin or hematocrit value.
- Maintain problem list, making appropriate plans and, if necessary, referrals.

12 MONTHS OF AGE

History (interim details)

- Assess parental concerns.
- Reassess social and system review.

Development

By this age:

- Gross motor:
  85% will cruise.
  70% will stand alone briefly.
  50% will walk to some extent, and more will try it with hands held.
- Fine motor:
  90% will bang two cubes together.
  70% will have a good pincer grasp.
- Language:
  80% will use "mama," "dada" specifically.
  30% will use as many as three additional words.
  Almost all will indulge in immature jargoning.
- Psychosocial:
  Almost all will respond to parent's presence and voice.
  Almost all will wave bye-bye.
  85% will play pat-a-cake.
  50% will drink from a cup.
  About half, perhaps a bit more, will play ball with examiner.

Physical Examination (particular attention)

- Update growth curves.
- Continue reassessment.
- Evaluate gait if walking has begun.

Anticipatory Guidance

- Reduced food intake in many (this is expected)
- Weaning or eliminating bottle use (especially at night)
- Increased use of table food
- Dental health, toothbrushing
- Toilet training (expectations, attitudes)
- Discipline (e.g., limit setting)
- Safety (childproofing house, car, neighborhood, etc.)

Plans and Problems

- Review immunizations, and provide as appropriate.

- Consider need for a serum lead level, hemoglobin or hematocrit value, tuberculosis testing.
- Maintain problem list, making appropriate plans and, if necessary, referrals.

15 MONTHS OF AGE

History (interim details)

- Assess parental concerns.
- Reassess social and system review.

Development

By this age:

- Gross motor:
  Almost all will walk well.
  Almost all will stoop to recover an object.
  35% will walk up steps with help.
- Fine motor:
  Almost all will drink from a cup.
  Almost all will have a neat pincer grasp.
  70% will scribble with crayon.
  60% will make a tower with two cubes.
- Language:
  Almost all will use "mama" and "dada" specifically.
  75% will use as many as three additional words.
  30% will put two words together.
- Psychosocial:
  Many more than 50% will play ball with examiner.
  50% will try to use a spoon.
  45% will try to remove clothing.

Physical Examination (particular attention)

- Update growth curves.
- Continue reassessment.
- Evaluate gait.

Anticipatory Guidance

- Negativism and independence
- Dental health (visit to a dentist)
- Toilet training
- Weaning
- Discipline (e.g., need for consistency)
- Safety (all issues, repetitively)

Plans and Problems
- Review immunizations, and provide as appropriate.
- Consider need for a serum lead level, hemoglobin or hematocrit value, tuberculosis testing.
- Maintain problem list, making appropriate plans and, if necessary, referrals.

18 MONTHS OF AGE

History (interim details)
- Assess parental concerns.
- Reassess social and system review.

Development

By this age:
- Gross motor:
  55% will have begun to walk up stairs without much help.
  70% will have started to walk backward.
  More than that will have tried running with at least some success.
  45% will have tried with some success to kick a ball forward, given the opportunity.
- Fine motor:
  80% will scribble if given a crayon.
  80% will make a tower with two cubes.
  About half of those will attempt, with some success, a tower of as many as four cubes.
- Language:
  Almost all will have mature jargoning.
  85% will have at least three words in addition to "mama" and "dada."
  Many of those will put two words together.
  More than half will respond to a one-step command (e.g., when asked to point to a body part).
- Psychosocial:
  Well more than half will assist with taking off their clothes.
  75% will use a spoon successfully, albeit with some spillage.

Physical Examination (particular attention)
- Update growth curves.
- Continue reassessment; search for new findings.
- Continue to evaluate gait.

Anticipatory Guidance
- Sleep (location, naps, nightmares)

- Diet (mealtime battles)
- Dental health (toothbrushing, dentist)
- Toilet training
- Discipline (methods and, again, consistency)
- Safety (never enough discussion [e.g., car seat, childproofing home])
- Self-comforting (masturbation, thumb sucking, favorite blankets and toys)
- Childcare settings if one is necessary

Plans and Problems

- Review immunizations, and provide as appropriate.
- Perform developmental and autism screening (using parent-administered validated tools).
- Consider need for serum lead level, hemoglobin or hematocrit value, tuberculosis testing.
- Maintain problem list, making appropriate plans and, if necessary, referrals.

2 YEARS OF AGE

History (interim details)

- Assess parental concerns.
- Reassess social and system review.

Development

By this age:

- Gross motor:
  All should run well.
  All should walk up steps of reasonable height without holding on.
  90% will kick a ball forward.
  80% will throw a ball overhand.
  60% will do a little jump.
  40% may balance on one foot for 1 to 2 seconds.
- Fine motor:
  Almost all should scribble with a pencil.
  90% will make a tower of four cubes.
  70% will copy a vertical line.
- Language:
  All should point to and name parts of body.
  85% will readily combine two different words.
  80% will understand "on," "under."
  75% will name a picture.

- Psychosocial:
  85% will give a toy to mother or other significant person.
  60% will put on some clothing alone and, often, also remove a
    garment.
  50% will play games with others.

Physical Examination (particular attention)
- Update growth curves.
- Continue reassessment; note new findings.
- Examine mouth, and count number of teeth.

Anticipatory Guidance
- Independence (limit setting, temper tantrums)
- Peer interaction
- Safety (poisons and potential poisons, water temperature, car seat use)
- Toilet training
- Nightmares
- Use of a cup for drinking (as much as possible)

Plans and Problems
- Review immunizations, and provide as appropriate.
- Perform developmental screening (using parent-administered validated tool).
- Consider need for serum lead level, hemoglobin or hematocrit value, dental referral, tuberculosis testing.
- Maintain problem list, making appropriate plans and, if necessary, referrals.

3 YEARS OF AGE
History (interim details)
- Assess parental concerns.
- Reassess social and system review.

Development
By this age:
- Gross motor:
  75% will balance on one foot for at least 1 second.
  75% will negotiate a successful broad jump.
  40% will balance on one foot for as long as 5 seconds.

- Fine motor:
  80% will copy a circle in addition to a vertical line.
  80% will build a tower of as many as eight cubes.
- Language:
  Speech is becoming more clearly understood in more than half.
  80% will use plurals appropriately.
  Almost half will give their first and last names appropriately.
- Psychosocial:
  90% will put on clothing alone.
  75% will play interactive games.
  50% will separate from mother or other significant person without
     too much stress.
  Many will have begun to wash and dry hands.

Physical Examination (particular attention)

- Update growth curves.
- Continue reassessment; note new findings.
- Assess whether teeth are coming in appropriately.

Anticipatory Guidance

- Degrees of independence (limit setting and encouragement, a fine
  balance), other aspects of discipline
- Safety (car seat, guns in the home, strangers)
- Personal hygiene (handwashing, toothbrushing, proper use of toi-
  let tissue)
- Daycare

Plans and Problems

- Review immunizations, and provide as appropriate.
- Perform developmental screening (using parent-administered vali-
  dated tool).
- Conduct formal vision screening.
- Consider need for serum lead level, hemoglobin or hematocrit
  value, tuberculosis testing.
- Maintain problem list, making appropriate plans and, if necessary,
  referrals.

4 YEARS OF AGE

History (interim details)

- Assess parental concerns.
- Reassess social and system review.

Development

By this age:

- Gross motor:
  75% will hop on one foot.
  75% will balance on one foot for as long as 5 seconds.
  65% will be able to imitate a heel-toe walk.
  Many will have begun to throw overhand.
- Fine motor:
  Almost all will copy a circle and a plus sign.
  80% will pick longer line of two.
  50% will begin to draw a person in three parts.
- Language:
  Speech is quite understandable in almost all.
  95% will give their first and last names.
  85% will understand "cold," "tired," "hungry."
  80% will identify three of four colors.
- Psychosocial:
  Almost all will play games with other children.
  70% will dress without supervision.

Physical Examination (particular attention)

- Update growth curves.
- Continue reassessment; note new findings.
- Remind that hearing and vision must be evaluated at each visit.
- Remind that taking blood pressure is an integral part of physical examination.

Anticipatory Guidance

- Importance of reading to child frequently
- Need for a booster seat in the car
- Fears and fantasies
- Separation (reliance on other adults as time goes by)
- Safety (matches and lighters out of reach, strangers, street, window guards)
- Personal hygiene (again, importance of frequent toothbrushing)

Plans and Problems

- Review immunizations, and provide as appropriate.
- Conduct formal hearing and vision screening.
- Consider need for serum lead level, hemoglobin or hematocrit value.
- Maintain problem list, making appropriate plans and, if necessary, referrals.

5 YEARS OF AGE

History (interim details)

- Assess parental concerns.
- Reassess social and system review.

Development

By this age:

- Gross motor:
  Almost all will hop nicely on one foot.
  75% will balance on one foot for as long as 10 seconds.
  60% will do a heel-toe walk backward reasonably well.
- Fine motor:
  85% will draw a person in three parts.
  65% will draw a person in as many as six parts.
  60% will copy a square.
- Language:
  Almost all will identify four colors.
  Almost all will understand "on," "under," "in front of," "behind."
  More than half will define adequately five of the following eight words—ball, cake, desk, house, banana, curtain, fence, ceiling.
- Psychosocial:
  Almost all will dress without supervision.
  Almost all will brush teeth without help.
  Almost all will play board and card games.
  Almost all will be relaxed when left with a babysitter.
  More than half will prepare their own cereal.

Physical Examination (particular attention)

- Update growth curves.
- Continue reassessment; note new findings.

Anticipatory Guidance

- Reading together
- School readiness (plays with others, endures separation from parents)
- Chores
- Discipline (consistency, praising)
- Gender identity
- Peer interaction
- Television
- Safety (booster seat, guns in home, bike helmets, pool safety)

  It is not usually possible to cover so many topics at one visit, so it is usually necessary to be selective based on your knowledge of the family situation.

Plans and Problems

- Review immunizations, and provide as appropriate.
- Consider need for tuberculosis testing.
- Maintain problem list, making appropriate plans and, if necessary, referrals.

ELEMENTARY SCHOOL YEARS (6-12 YEARS OF AGE)

History (interim details)

- Parental concerns
- Child's concerns
- Reassess social and system review
- Attention span
- Behavior at home and in school
- School accomplishments and experience
- Enuresis, encopresis, constipation, nightmares

Development

By this time, gross and fine motor problems have most often become apparent (but not always; neurologic examination should not be short-changed). Language and psychosocial skills can be readily investigated in talks with parents and child and in explorations of school and play experiences. Socialization and developing maturity may have different expressions at home, on the playground, and in school, and when with people of different ages and different degrees of acquaintance. Talks with teachers, report cards, and various drawings and other efforts that the child brings home from school can be very helpful.

Physical Examination (particular attention)

- Update growth curves.
- Continue reassessment; note new findings.
- Begin Tanner stage assessment.

Anticipatory Guidance

- Parent–child rapport
- Need for praise
- Responsibility
- Safety (booster seat and seat belt use, guns in the home, fire safety, bike helmets, pool safety)
- Allowance
- Television
- Sex education

- Dental care
- Adult supervision
- Discipline (limit setting)

Again, time constraints almost always make it necessary to adjust the menu for anticipatory guidance to your judgment about the family's needs.

Plans and Problems

- Review immunizations, and provide as appropriate.
- Consider need for tuberculosis testing.
- Consider dyslipidemia screening.
- Maintain problem list, making appropriate plans and, if necessary, referrals.

ADOLESCENTS

We have assumed a continuing relationship with the patient from birth on. If you are seeing a patient for the first time, begin with a full history and physical examination.

History (interim details)

- Patient's concerns
- Parental concerns
- Menstrual history
- Use of tobacco, alcohol, recreational drugs
- Diet and exercise
- Sexual activity (relationships, partner violence, pregnancy and contraceptive use); exact timing for all of this should rely on your assessment of the situation and your judgment; in general, social experience
- School experience
- Suicidal ideation; always be on the alert, and bring it up when necessary
- Update knowledge of home and family structure

An adolescent patient (and some elementary-school children) may prefer to be or should be seen alone at times and as they get older, most often or always. This does not mean, however, that the parents are not involved. Proper balance in this relies on your judgment.

Development

By this time adolescent's physical, neurologic, and cognitive abilities should be well understood, but nothing should be taken for granted.

Conversation with patient, parent or parents, and teachers; school records; and, of course, a careful physical examination should all be helpful.

Physical Examination (particular attention)

- Update growth curves.
- Continue reassessment; note new findings.
- Tanner stage assessment.
- Assess spinal curvatures, particularly in early-adolescent female patients.

Anticipatory Guidance

- Puberty and its issues; body image
- Sexuality, gender identity, sexually transmitted infections, contraception
- Diet
- Tobacco, alcohol, drugs
- Risk-taking behavior
- Exercise
- Safety (guns in the home, seat-belt use, bike helmets)
- Family and other social relationships
- Independence and responsibility
- School and the future

Time constraints almost always make it necessary to adjust the menu for anticipatory guidance to your judgment about the adolescent's and/or the family's needs.

Plans and Problems

- Review immunizations, and provide as appropriate.
- Consider need for tuberculosis testing, sexually transmitted infection screening, hemoglobin or hematocrit determination, dyslipidemia screening.
- Maintain problem list, making appropriate plans and, if necessary, referrals.

22 Age-Specific Examination: Special Populations and Older Adults

Examination Guidelines

Variability exists in knowledge, experience, cognitive abilities, and personality among patients. These differences can affect your interaction. Persons with disabilities and older adults may experience some decline in their abilities, and these changes may not all occur at the same rate. Adaptation to patients' needs with disabling physical, intellectual, or emotional states (e.g., acute disabling illness, deafness, blindness, depression, psychosis, developmental delays, or neurologic impairments) is necessary.

Interviewing a patient with a physical disability. Note the uncluttered surroundings; be sure the patient in a wheelchair has room to maneuver.

Some patients have sensory losses, such as hearing, that make communication more difficult. Position yourself so that the patient can see your face. Speak clearly and slowly; shouting magnifies the problem by distorting consonants and vowels. For deaf patients who use sign language, use of a sign language interpreter is best. Impaired vision and difficulties with light–dark adaptation are a problem with written interview forms. Large print and lighting that does not glare or reflect in the eyes or individualized assistance is helpful.

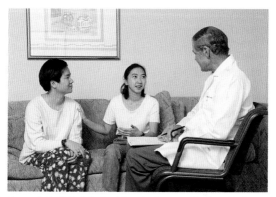

Interviewing a patient with the help of an interpreter. Someone other than a family member should act as interpreter to bridge the language difference between the health care provider and the patient.

The patient has most often learned the best way to be transferred from a wheelchair or bed to another site or to a different position. Consult patient about this.

Let a hearing-, speech-, or vision-impaired patient guide you to the best communication system for your mutual purposes.

Bowel and bladder concerns are common to many individuals with disabilities and should be given the necessary attention during the examination process.

COGNITIVE ASSESSMENT

Some older adults or individuals with intellectual disability may be confused or experience memory loss, particularly for recent events. Take whatever extra time is needed. Ask short (but not leading) questions, and keep your language simple. Consult other family members to clarify discrepancies or to fill in the gaps. When necessary, use other health care professionals involved in care and the patient's record as resources for a more complete background.

Mental status is assessed continuously throughout the entire interaction with a patient by evaluating the patient's alertness, orientation, cognitive abilities, and mood. Observe the patient's physical appearance, behavior, and responses to questions asked during the history (see figure on next page). Evaluate the patient's mental status throughout the encounter (see Chapter 3).

During the initial greeting, observe the patient for behavior, emotional status, grooming, and body language. Note the patient's body posture and ability to make eye contact.

TESTING MEMORY IN VISUALLY IMPAIRED PATIENTS

When a patient is visually impaired, test recent memory with unrelated words rather than observed objects. Pick four unrelated words that sound distinctly different, such as "green," "daffodil," "hero," and "sofa" or "bird," "carpet," "treasure," and "orange." Tell the patient to remember these words. After 5 minutes, ask the patient to list the four words.

Cognitive impairment that deprives ability to join in decision-making processes underscores the need for advance directives, which document the patient's wishes regarding extraordinary means of life support (e.g., ventilation assistance and feeding tubes). This document should be complemented by a surrogate (e.g., spouse, child, sibling, or other person with a close relationship) who has a legally executed durable power of attorney for health care.

Multiple health conditions that require multiple medications increase risk for iatrogenic disorders and issues related to interactions. A medication history with attention to interactions of drugs, diseases, and aging is needed for prescribed and over-the-counter medications and herbal preparations.

Aging, disability, a debilitating illness, and the onset of frailty increase dependency on others, worry about tomorrow, and grieving for what has been lost. Recognize these vast concerns and the sense of loss in both the patient and the immediate caregiver. Maintaining function is a compelling concern of older adults.

FUNCTIONAL ASSESSMENT

Functional assessment is an evaluation of a patient's ability to achieve the basic activities of daily living (ADLs). Questions concerning the ability to take care of one's daily needs are part of the review of systems.

Activities of Daily Living

The ability to perform instrumental ADLs, or the ability to live independently, is an important assessment. Determine the patient's ability to perform the following:

ADLs Assessment

Shop, cook, and prepare nutritious meals.
Use problem-solving skills.
Manage medications (purchase, understand, and follow directions).
Manage personal finances and business affairs.
Speak, write, and understand spoken and written language.
Remember appointments, family occasions, holidays, and household tasks.

The personal and social history should include other dimensions of functional capacity such as social, spiritual, and economic resources; recreational activity; sleep patterns; environmental control; and use of the health care system.

Functional assessment should be performed for anyone limited by disease or disability and includes:

Functional Assessment

MOBILITY	UPPER EXTREMITY FUNCTION
Difficulty walking standard distances: 1/2 mile, 2 to 3 blocks, 1/3 block, across a room	Difficulty grasping small objects, opening jars
Difficulty climbing stairs, up and down	Difficulty reaching out or up overhead, such as to take something off a shelf
Problems with balance	
Housework	**Instrumental ADLs**
Heavy (vacuuming, scrubbing floors)	Bathing
Light (dusting)	Dressing
Meal preparation	Toileting
Shopping	Moving from bed to chair, chair to standing
	Eating
	Walking in home

Any limitations will affect a patient's independence and autonomy, and increase reliance on other people and on assistive devices.

In older patients, these limitations indicate the loss of physical reserve and the potential loss of physical function and independence that indicate the onset of frailty.

Characteristics of Frailty

Unintentional weight loss of 5% or more in past year	Weak grip strength
Unable to walk up a flight of steps	Low activity
Feeling of exhaustion	Increased number of illnesses

Frailty is an at-risk state caused by the age-associated accumulation of deficits resulting from cardiovascular and respiratory diseases and diabetes. Identification is important because of its association with functional decline, disability, and poor health outcomes (Phillips-Burkhart, 2016).

The Healthy Female Evaluation

The following are items to consider for inclusion as part of a routine female health examination or well-woman visit. This is not intended as an all-inclusive list. Some items may vary depending on the patient's age, health status, and particular risk factors. Medical history and review of systems may also be indicated. Age and risk-status guidelines for preventive services are available from a variety of sources and authorities.*

History

HISTORY OF PRESENT ILLNESS
- Age
- Last normal menstrual period
- Menopause—age achieved, symptoms
- Obstetric history—number of pregnancies, term pregnancies, preterm pregnancies, abortions/miscarriages, living children (GTPAL)
- Contraceptive measures and history
- Sexual history
- Breast lumps, discharge, pain, skin changes
- Unusual vaginal bleeding or discharge
- Abdominal or pelvic pain or bloating
- Urinary symptoms

RISK ASSESSMENT
- Cardiovascular—smoking, hypertension, diet, body mass index (BMI), exercise, family history
- Cancer—personal/family history of breast, ovarian, or colon cancer; history of sun exposure
- Infection—sexually transmitted infection (STI) exposure; tuberculosis exposure; hepatitis i exposure; Immunizations:
  - tetanus/flu – all ages
  - HPV - before age 26 years

---

*Authorities that produce prevention guidelines include Academy of Family Physicians, American Cancer Society, American College of Obstetricians and Gynecologists, American College of Physicians, American Geriatrics Society, Canadian Task Force on the Periodic Health Examination, National Cancer Institute, and U.S. Preventive Services Task Force.

- pneumonia - age 65 years and older
- herpes zoster (shingles) - age 60 years and older
- Metabolic—calcium supplement, family/personal history of osteoporosis; exercise; personal/family history of diabetes mellitus; hearing impairment in older adults
- Injury—alcohol, seat belts, guns, family/partner violence
- Mental health—depression: vegetative symptoms (eating, sleeping, concentration, energy, social interaction)

HEALTH HABITS

- Breast self-awareness
- Pap smear—date, result of last Pap smear; any abnormal, treatment
- Human papillomavirus (HPV) test—date, result of last test
- Mammogram—date, result of last mammogram
- Diet—proportion of fat, protein, carbohydrate; calcium, vitamin D
- Exercise—amount, frequency
- Smoking/tobacco use—type, amount, frequency
- Alcohol/drug use—type, amount, frequency

Physical Examination

- Vital signs: blood pressure
- Height and weight; BMI
- Skin—lesions, moles
- Respiratory—rate, pattern, additional sounds
- Cardiovascular—rate, rhythm, regularity, additional sounds
- Peripheral vascular—pulses, edema, clubbing
- Breasts—contour, masses, nipple discharge, skin changes
- Lymph—regional lymphadenopathy (infraclavicular and supraclavicular, axillary, inguinal)
- Abdomen—bowel sounds, masses, organ enlargement, hernias
- Pelvic—lesions, discharge; Bartholin glands, urethra, Skene glands; vagina, cervix, adnexa, uterus; rectovaginal septum
- Rectal—hemorrhoids, masses, lesions

Screening Recommendations

- Cardiovascular
  Blood pressure—begin at age 18
  Lipid profile—begin at age 45
- Cancer

Cervical: Pap smear/HPV testing:

- Ages 21 to 29 years: Pap test every 3 years. HPV testing should not be used in this age group unless it is needed after an abnormal Pap test result.
- Ages 30 to 65 years: Pap test plus an HPV test every 5 years or Pap test alone every 3 years.
- Patients older than 65 years at average risk who have had regular cervical cancer testing with normal results testing not recommended. Once testing is stopped, it should not be started again. Patients with a history of a serious cervical precancer (cervical intraepithelial neoplasia grade 2 or 3) should continue with routine testing for at least 20 years after diagnosis, even if testing continues past age 65 years.
- Patients with uterus and cervix removed for reasons not related to cervical cancer and who have no history of cervical cancer or serious precancer should not be tested.
- Patients vaccinated against HPV should follow the screening recommendations for her age group.

Breast

- Clinical breast examination—younger than 40 years: every 3 years; older than 40 years: annually
- Screening mammogram—annually beginning at age 40 years; earlier if at increased risk; frequency depends on personal and family history and past results

Colorectal: begin age 50 years. Options are:

- Tests that detect adenomatous polyps and cancer:
  - Flexible sigmoidoscopy every 5 years
  - Colonoscopy every 10 years
  - Double-contrast barium enema every 5 years
  - Computed tomography colography every 5 years
- Tests that primarily detect cancer:
  - Annual guaiac-based fecal occult blood test with high test sensitivity
  - Annual fecal immunochemical test with high test sensitivity
  - Stool DNA test with high sensitivity (testing interval uncertain)

Lung

- Ages 55 to 80 years: annual screening with low-dose computed tomography (LDCT) in those who have a 30 pack-year smoking history and currently smoke or have quit within the past 15 years. Screening should be discontinued once a person has not smoked for 15 years or develops a health problem that substantially limits life expectancy or the ability or willingness to have curative lung surgery.

- Infection

  STI testing—depending on exposure status; chlamydia screening—all sexually active women age 25 years or younger and women older than age 25 years with risk factors (e.g., women with a new or more than one sex partner); gonorrhea and syphilis screening—all sexually active women at increased risk

  TB skin testing—depending on risk status

- Metabolic

  BMI: obesity

  Fasting plasma glucose for those ages 40 to 70 years who are overweight or obese

  Bone density—women ≥65 years; begin earlier in women whose fracture risk is equal to or greater than that of a 65-year-old white woman who has no additional risk factors

  Hearing impairment—older adults

- Injury

  Intimate partner violence (see Appendix A: Quick Reference to Special Histories)

- Mental health

  Alcohol and substance abuse (see Appendix A: Quick Reference to Special Histories)

  Depression

Sports Participation Evaluation

The overall goal of the preparticipation physical evaluation (PPE) is to ensure safe participation in an appropriate physical activity and not to restrict participation unnecessarily. Whether athletes receive the PPE in the context of an ongoing primary care relationship or as a focused preseason checkup, the following goals of the evaluation are universal:

- To identify conditions that may interfere with a person's ability to participate in a sport
- To identify health problems that increase the risk for injury or death during sports participation
- To help select an appropriate sport for a person's particular abilities and physical status

Sports and disciplined physical effort enhance fitness and coordination, increase self-esteem, and provide positive social experiences for participants, including individuals with physical and intellectual disabilities. Few children and youth have conditions that might limit participation, and most of these conditions are known before the PPE takes place. The PPE should be completed 6 weeks before or well enough in advance of the planned sports activity so that any needed specialist evaluations, rehabilitation, or therapy can be completed before participation begins.

Examination Guidelines

Recommended components of the PPE include a focused medical history and examinations of high-yield areas, like the cardiac and orthopedic systems. Important physical examination items follow history items in the following box.

Recommended Components of the Preparticipation Physical Evaluation (PPE)

History
General Medical History
- Illnesses or injuries since the last health visit or PPE
- History of having been denied or restricted from participation in sporting activities and reason for restriction

Continued

Recommended Components of the Preparticipation Physical Evaluation (PPE)—cont'd

- History of heat illness or muscle cramps
- Current viral illness (patients with mononucleosis may return to play after 3 weeks if no longer symptomatic and no splenomegaly; fever at the time of the exam is an absolute contraindication because of the association with viral myocarditis)
- Sickle cell trait or disease (adequate hydration is necessary and caution should be taken to avoid extreme conditions due to risk of rhabdomyolysis)
- Hospitalizations or surgeries
- All medications used by the athlete (including steroids and nutritional supplements or medications taken to enhance performance)
- Use of any special equipment or protective devices during sports participation
- Allergies (including food-, insect bite–, and exercise-provoked allergies), particularly those associated with anaphylaxis or respiratory compromise
- Absence of paired organs (single-organ athletes may participate if the single organ can be protected and the patient/caregivers understand the risks involved)
- Immunization status, including hepatitis B, varicella, meningococcal, human papillomavirus, and pertussis

Cardiac
- Symptoms of exertional chest pain/discomfort
- Unexplained syncope or near-syncope
- Excessive exertional and unexplained dyspnea/fatigue, associated with exercise
- Prior recognition of a heart murmur
- Family history of premature death (sudden and unexpected, or otherwise) before age 50 years as a result of heart disease in one or more relatives
- Family history of disability from heart disease in a close relative younger than 50 years
- Specific knowledge of certain cardiac conditions in family members: hypertrophic or dilated cardiomyopathy, long-QT syndrome or other ion channelopathies, Marfan syndrome, or clinically important arrhythmias

Respiratory
- Coughing, wheezing, or dyspnea with exercise
- Previous use of asthma medications
- Family history of asthma

Neurologic
- History of a head injury with or without symptoms of a concussion (confusion, prolonged headache, memory problems)

Recommended Components of the Preparticipation Physical Evaluation (PPE)—cont'd

- Numbness or tingling in the extremities
- Headaches
- History of seizure
- History of inability to move an extremity after a collision

Vision
- Visual problems
- Glasses or contact lenses
- Previous eye injuries

Orthopedic
- Previous injuries that have limited sports practice or participation
- Injuries that have been associated with pain, swelling, or the need for medical intervention
- Previous fractures or dislocated joints
- Previous or current use of a brace, orthotic, or other assistive device

Psychosocial
- Weight control and body image
- Dietary habits, calcium intake
- Stresses in personal life, at home, or in school
- Feelings of sadness, hopelessness, depression, or anxiety
- Use or abuse of recreational drugs, alcohol, tobacco, or dietary or performance supplements

Genitourinary and Abdominal
- Age at menarche, last menstrual period, regularity of menstrual periods, number of periods in the last year, and longest interval between periods (athletic girls tend to experience menarche at a later age than nonathletic girls).

Dermatologic
- History of rashes, pressure sores, or other skin conditions
- History of boils or methicillin-resistant *Staphylococcus aureus* (MRSA) skin infections

Physical Examination
General
- Height, weight, and body mass index (BMI)
- Palpation of lymph nodes
- Attention to signs of eating disorders, including oral ulcerations, decreased tooth enamel, edema

Continued

Recommended Components of the Preparticipation Physical Evaluation (PPE)—cont'd

Cardiac and Pulses
- Elevated systemic blood pressure
- Heart murmur (auscultation should be performed in both supine and standing positions, or with Valsalva maneuver, to identify murmurs of dynamic left ventricular outflow obstruction); heart rate and rhythm to assess for arrhythmias
- Femoral pulses to exclude coarctation of the aorta
- Brachial artery blood pressure (sitting position with appropriate size cuff, preferably taken in both arms)

Respiratory
- Lung auscultation

Neurologic
- Comprehensive neurologic exam

Vision
- Visual acuity

Orthopedic
- Screening orthopedic examination
- Physical stigmata of Marfan syndrome (e.g., arm span greater than height and hyperextensible joints)

Genitourinary and Abdominal
- Palpation of the abdomen for organomegaly
- Palpation of the testicles for masses
- Examination for inguinal hernias

Dermatologic
- Skin lesions suggestive of herpes simplex virus (HSV), MRSA, or tinea corporis

Modified from Andrews, 1997; Maron et al, 2015; and 2010 Preparticipation Physical Evaluation History and Physical Examination Forms endorsed by the American Academy of Family Physicians, American Academy of Pediatrics, American College of Sports Medicine, American Medical Society for Sports Medicine, American Orthopedic Society for Sports Medicine, and the American Osteopathic Academy of Sports Medicine. Forms are publicly available at: https://www.aap.org/en-us/about-the-aap/Committees-Councils-Sections/Council-on-sports-medicine-and-fitness/.

Garrick's "2-minute" 14-step orthopedic screening examination consists of observing the athlete in a variety of positions and postures that highlight asymmetries in range of motion, strength, and muscle bulk. These asymmetries serve to identify acute or old, poorly rehabilitated injuries. The steps shown in the figure on pp. 306-307 help in assessing most of the following:

- Posture and general muscle contour bilaterally
- Patient's duck walk, four steps with knees completely bent
- Spine for curvature and lumbar extension, fingers touching toes with knees straight
- Shoulder and clavicle for dislocation
- Neck, shoulders, elbows, forearms, hands, fingers, and hips for range of motion
- Knee ligaments for drawer sign

You should also assess the following:

- Gait
- Patient's ability to hop on each foot
- Patient's ability to walk on tiptoes and heels

Once a PPE has been completed, the health care provider can guide the patient with sport selection, plan therapy or rehabilitation of conditions or injuries, and in rare instances, discuss restrictions. The clinician may: (1) provide "clearance" for participation, (2) provide "clearance" for participation with recommendations for further evaluation and/or treatment, (3) restrict participation until further testing is performed, or (4) recommend complete restriction from specific sports or all sports. Decisions are made at the discretion of the clinician, but recommendations to limit participation are not legally binding. Patients with findings from the PPE may require evaluation by a health care provider with appropriate knowledge and experience to assess the safety of a given sport for the athlete.

Step 3: Have the athlete shrug the shoulders against resistance from the examiner to evaluate trapezius strength.

Step 1: Observe the standing athlete from the front for symmetry of trunk, shoulders, and extremities.

Step 2: Observe neck flexion, extension, lateral flexion on each side, and rotation to evaluate range of motion and the cervical spine.

Step 4: Have the athlete perform shoulder abduction against resistance from the examiner to assess deltoid strength.

Step 5: Observe internal and external rotation of the shoulder to evaluate range of motion of the glenohumeral joint.

Step 6: Observe extension and flexion of the elbow to assess range of motion.

Step 7: Observe pronation and supination of the forearm to evaluate elbow and wrist range of motion.

Step 8: Have the athlete clench the fist, then spread the fingers to assess range of motion in the hand and fingers.

Step 9: Observe the standing athlete from the rear for symmetry of trunk, shoulders, and extremities.

Step 10: Have the athlete stand with the knees straight and bend backward from the waist. Discomfort with extension of the lumbar spine may be associated with spondylolysis and spondylolisthesis.

Step 11: Have the athlete stand with the knees straight and flex forward at the waist, first away from the examiner, then toward the examiner, to assess for scoliosis, spine range of motion, and hamstring flexibility.

Step 12: Have the athlete stand facing the examiner with quadriceps flexed to observe symmetry of leg musculature.

Step 13: Have the athlete duck walk four steps to assess hip, knee, and ankle range of motion, strength, and balance.

Step 14: Have the athlete stand on the toes, then the heels to evaluate calf strength, symmetry, and balance.

The 14-step screening orthopedic examination. The athlete should be dressed so that the joints and muscle groups included in the examination are easily visible: usually gym shorts for males and gym shorts and a T-shirt for females. Keep in mind that one of the most important points to look for in the orthopedic screening examination is symmetry.

25 Documentation

Subjective Data—The History

Subjective data are the positive and negative pieces of information that the patient offers. Record the patient's history, especially during an initial visit, to provide a comprehensive database. Arrange information appropriately in specific categories, usually in a particular sequence such as chronologic order with most recent information first. Include both positive and negative data that contribute to the assessment. Use the following organized sequence as a guide.

IDENTIFYING INFORMATION

Record data recommended by the health care facility.
- Patient's name
- Identification number/social security number
- Age, sex
- Marital status
- Address (home and business)
- Phone numbers
- Occupation, employer
- Insurance plan, number
- Date of visit
- For children and dependent adults, names of parents or next of kin
  Put identifying information on each page of record.

SOURCE AND RELIABILITY OF INFORMATION
- Document who is providing the history and relationship to patient.
- Indicate when an old record is used.
- State judgment about reliability of information.

CHIEF CONCERN/PRESENTING PROBLEM/REASON FOR SEEKING CARE

Record a description of the patient's main reasons for seeking health care, in patient's own words with quotation marks. Paraphrase only if this makes the patient's concern more clear. Include duration of problem.

HISTORY OF PRESENT PROBLEM

- List and describe current symptoms of chief concern and their appearance chronologically in reverse order, dating events and symptoms.
- List any expected symptoms that are absent.
- Identify anyone in household with same symptoms.
- Note pertinent information from review of systems, family history, and personal/social history along with findings.
- Where more than one problem is identified, address each in a separate paragraph, including the following details of symptom occurrence:
  - Onset: when problem first started, chronologic order of events, setting and circumstances, manner of onset (sudden versus gradual)
  - Location: exact location, localized or generalized, radiation patterns
  - Duration: how long problem has lasted, intermittent or continuous, duration of each episode
  - Character: nature of symptom
  - Aggravating/associated factors: food, activity, rest, certain movements; nausea, vomiting, diarrhea, fever, chills, etc.
  - Relieving factors: prescribed treatments and/or self-remedies, alternative or complementary therapies, their effect on the problem; food, rest, heat, ice, activity, position, etc.
  - Temporal factors: frequency; relation to other symptoms, problems, functions; symptom improvement or worsening over time
  - Severity of symptoms: quantify on a 0 (minimal) to 10 (severe) scale; effect on patient's lifestyle

MEDICAL HISTORY

- List and describe each of the following with dates of occurrence and any specific information available:
  - General health and strength over lifetime as patient perceives it; disabilities and functional limitations
  - Hospitalization and/or surgery: dates, hospital, diagnosis, complications
  - Injuries and disabilities
  - Major childhood illnesses
  - Adult illnesses and serious injuries

- Immunizations: polio, diphtheria-pertussis-tetanus, tetanus toxoid, *Haemophilus influenza* type b, hepatitis A and B, measles, mumps, rubella, varicella, Prevnar, influenza, anthrax, smallpox, cholera, typhus, typhoid, meningococcal, pneumococcal, bacille Calmette-Guérin, last purified protein derivative or other skin tests, unusual reaction to immunizations
- Medications: past, current, recent medications (prescribed, nonprescription, complementary therapies, home remedies); dosages
- Allergies: drugs, foods, environmental
- Transfusions: reason, date, number of units transfused, reactions
- Emotional status: history of mood disorders, psychiatric attention, or medications
- Recent laboratory tests (e.g., glucose, cholesterol, Pap smear, mammogram, prostate-specific antigen)

Family History

- Present information about age and health of family members in narrative or pedigree form, including at least three generations.
- Family members: Include parents, grandparents, aunts and uncles, siblings, spouse, children. For deceased family members, note age at time of death and cause, if known.
- Major health or genetic disorders: Include hypertension; cancer; cardiac, respiratory, kidney, or thyroid disorders; strokes; asthma or other allergic manifestations; blood dyscrasia; psychiatric difficulties; tuberculosis; diabetes mellitus; hepatitis; or other familial disorders. Note spontaneous abortions and stillbirths.

PERSONAL/SOCIAL HISTORY

- Include information according to concerns of patient and influence of health problem on patient's and family's life:
  - Cultural background and practices, birthplace, position in family
  - Marital status
  - Religious preference, religious or cultural proscriptions for medical care
  - Home conditions: economic condition, number in household, pets, presence of smoke detectors, presence and security of firearms

- Occupation: work conditions and hours; physical or mental strain; protective devices used; exposure to chemicals, toxins, poisons, fumes, smoke, asbestos, or radioactive material at home or work
- Environment: home, school, work; structural barriers if handicapped, community services utilized; travel; exposure to contagious diseases
- Current health habits and/or risk factors: exercise; smoking; salt intake; weight control; dental hygiene diet, vitamins and other supplements; caffeine-containing beverages; alcohol or recreational drug use; response to CAGE, TACE, or CRAFFT questions (see Appendix A) related to alcohol use; participation in a drug or alcohol treatment program or support group
- Sexual activity: protection method, contraception
- General life satisfaction, hobbies, interests, sources of stress, adolescent's response to HEEADSSS questions (see Appendix)

REVIEW OF SYSTEMS

- Organize in general head-to-toe sequence, including an impression of each symptom.
- Record expected or negative findings as absence of symptoms or problems.
- When unexpected or positive findings are stated by patient, include details from further inquiry as you would in the present illness.
- Include the following categories of information (sequence may vary):
  - General constitutional symptoms
  - Diet
  - Skin, hair, nails
  - Head and neck
  - Eyes, ears, nose, mouth, throat
  - Endocrine
  - Breasts
  - Heart and blood vessels
  - Chest and lungs
  - Hematologic
  - Lymphatic and immunologic
  - Gastrointestinal
  - Genitourinary
  - Musculoskeletal
  - Neurologic
  - Psychiatric

Objective Data—Physical Findings

Objective data are the findings resulting from direct observation—what you see, hear, and touch.

GENERAL STATEMENT

- Age, race, sex, general appearance
- Nutritional status, weight, height, frame size, body mass index
- Vital signs: temperature, pulse rate, respiratory rate, blood pressure (two extremities, two positions)

MENTAL STATUS

- Physical appearance and behavior
- Cognitive: memory, reasoning, attention span, response to questions
- Speech and language: voice quality, articulation, content, coherence, comprehension
- Emotional stability: anxiety, depression, disturbance in thought content

SKIN

- Color, integrity, temperature, hydration, tattoos, scars
- Presence of edema, excessive perspiration, unusual odor
- Presence and description of lesions (size, shape, location, inflammation, tenderness, induration, discharge), parasites
- Hair texture and distribution
- Nail configuration, color, texture, condition, presence of clubbing, nail plate adherence, firmness

HEAD

- Size and contour of head, scalp appearance and movement
- Facial features (characteristics, symmetry)
- Presence of edema or puffiness, tenderness
- Temporal arteries: characteristics

EYES

- Visual acuity, visual fields
- Appearance of orbits, conjunctivae, sclerae, eyelids, eyebrows
- Pupillary shape, consensual response to light and accommodation, extraocular movements, corneal light reflex, cover–uncover test
- Ophthalmoscopic findings of cornea, lens, retina, optic disc, macula, retinal vessel size, caliber, and arteriovenous crossings

EARS

- Configuration, position and alignment of auricles
- Otoscopic findings of canals (cerumen, lesions, discharge, foreign body) and tympanic membranes (integrity, color, landmarks, mobility, perforation)
- Hearing: air and bone conduction tests, whispered voice, conversation

NOSE

- Appearance of external nose, nasal patency, flaring
- Nasal mucosa and septum, color, alignment, discharge, crusting, polyp
- Appearance of turbinates
- Presence of sinus tenderness or swelling
- Discrimination of odors

MOUTH AND THROAT

- Number, occlusion and condition of teeth; presence of dental appliances
- Lips, tongue, buccal and oral mucosa, floor of mouth (color, moisture, surface characteristics, ulcerations, induration, symmetry)
- Oropharynx, tonsils, palate (color, symmetry, exudate)
- Symmetry and movement of tongue, soft palate and uvula; gag reflex
- Discrimination of taste

NECK

- Mobility, suppleness, strength
- Position of trachea
- Thyroid size, shape, tenderness, nodules
- Presence of masses, webbing, skinfolds

CHEST

- Size and shape of chest, anteroposterior versus transverse diameter, symmetry of movement with respiration
- Presence of retractions, use of accessory muscles, diaphragmatic excursion

LUNGS

- Respiratory rate, depth, regularity, quietness or ease of respiration

- Palpation findings: symmetry and quality of tactile fremitus, thoracic expansion
- Percussion findings: quality and symmetry of percussion notes, diaphragmatic excursion
- Auscultation findings: characteristics of breath sounds (pitch, duration, intensity, vesicular, bronchial, bronchovesicular), unexpected breath sounds
- Characteristics of cough
- Presence of friction rub, egophony, whispered pectoriloquy

BREASTS

- Size, contour, venous patterns
- Symmetry, texture, masses, scars, tenderness, thickening, nodules, discharge, retraction, or dimpling
- Characteristics of nipples and areolae

HEART

- Anatomic location of apical impulse
- Heart rate, rhythm, amplitude, contour
- Palpation findings: pulsations, thrills, heaves, or lifts
- Auscultation findings: characteristics of S_1 and S_2 (location, intensity, pitch, timing, splitting, systole, diastole)
- Presence of murmurs, clicks, snaps, S_3 or S_4 (timing, location, radiation intensity, pitch, quality)

BLOOD VESSELS

- Blood pressure: comparison between extremities with position change
- Jugular vein pulsations and distention, pressure measurement
- Presence of bruits over carotid, temporal, renal, and femoral arteries, abdominal aorta
- Pulses in distal extremities
- Temperature, color, hair distribution, skin texture, nail beds of lower extremities
- Presence of edema, swelling, vein distention, Homans sign, or tenderness of lower extremities

ABDOMEN

- Shape, contour, visible aorta pulsations, venous patterns, hernia
- Auscultation findings: bowel sounds in all quadrants, character

- Palpation findings: aorta, organs, feces, masses, location, size, contour, consistency, tenderness, muscle resistance
- Percussion findings: areas of different percussion notes, costovertebral angle tenderness
- Liver span

FEMALE GENITALIA

- Appearance of external genitalia and perineum, distribution of pubic hair, inflammation, excoriation, tenderness, scarring, discharge
- Internal examination findings: appearance of vaginal mucosa, cervix, discharge, odor, lesions
- Bimanual examination findings: size, position, tenderness of cervix, vaginal walls, uterus, adnexa, ovaries
- Rectovaginal examination findings
- Urinary incontinence with bearing down

MALE GENITALIA

- Appearance of external genitalia, circumcision status, location and size of urethral opening, discharge, lesions, distribution of pubic hair
- Palpation findings: penis, testes, epididymides, vasa deferentia, contour, consistency, tenderness
- Presence of hernia or scrotal swelling

ANUS AND RECTUM

- Sphincter control, presence of hemorrhoids, fissures, skin tags, polyps
- Rectal wall contour, tenderness, sphincter tone
- Prostate size, contour, consistency, mobility
- Color and consistency of stool

LYMPHATIC

- Presence of lymph nodes in head, neck, epitrochlear, axillary, or inguinal areas
- Size, shape, consistency, warmth, tenderness, mobility, discreteness of nodes

MUSCULOSKELETAL

- Posture: Alignment of extremities and spine, symmetry of body parts

- Symmetry of muscle mass, tone and muscle strength; grading of strength, fasciculations, spasms
- Range of motion, passive and active; presence of pain with movement
- Appearance of joints; presence of deformities, effusions, warmth, tenderness, or crepitus

NEUROLOGIC
- Cranial nerves: specific findings for each or specify those tested, if findings are recorded in head and neck sections
- Cerebellar and motor function: gait, balance, coordination with rapid alternating motions
- Sensory function, symmetry (touch, pain, vibration, temperature, monofilament)
- Superficial and deep tendon reflexes: symmetry, grade

Assessment

The assessment section is composed of your interpretations and conclusions, their rationale, the diagnostic possibilities, and present and anticipated problems—what you think.

For each new and existing problem on the problem list, make a differential diagnosis list with rationale based on subjective and objective data. Describe disease progression or complication.

Plan

The plan describes the need to invoke diagnostic resources, therapeutic modalities, and other resources and the rationale for these decisions—what you intend to do.
- Diagnostic tests ordered or performed
- Therapeutic treatment plan
- Patient education
- Referrals initiated
- Future visit to evaluate plan

References

ACOG Committee on Adolescent Health Care: Human papillomavirus vaccination. Number 641. http://www.acog.org/Resources-And-Publications/Committee-Opinions/Committee-on-Adolescent-Health-Care/Human-Papillomavirus-Vaccination, 2015 (Accessed Sept 14, 2016).

American Academy of Pediatrics: HPV Champion Toolkit. https://www.aap.org/en-us/advocacy-and-policy/aap-health-initiatives/Pages/HPV-Champion-Toolkit, 2016 (Accessed Sept 16, 2016).

American Academy of Pediatrics: Male circumcision, *Pediatrics* 130(3):e756–e785, 2012. http://pediatrics.aappublications.org/content/130/3/585 (Accessed Oct 5, 2016).

American Cancer Society: Oral cavity and oropharyngeal cancers. http://www.cancer.org/Cancer/OralCavityandOropharyngealCancer/DetailedGuide/oral-cavity-and-oropharyngeal-cancer-risk-factors, 2016 (Accessed Nov 21, 2016).

American Cancer Society: Prostate cancer risk factors. http://www.cancer.org/cancer/prostatecancer/detailedguide/prostate-cancer-risk-factors, 2016 (Accessed Oct 6, 2016).

American Cancer Society: Risk factors for endometrial cancer. http://www.cancer.org/cancer/endometrialcancer/detailedguide/endometrial-uterine-cancer-risk-factors, 2016 (Accessed Oct 2, 2016).

American Cancer Society: The updated breast cancer screening guideline from the American Cancer Society. http://www.cancer.org/healthy/informationforhealthcareprofessionals/acsguidelines/breastcancerscreeningguidelines/index, 2015 (Accessed Oct 2, 2016).

American Cancer Society: What are the risk factors for anal cancer? http://www.cancer.org/cancer/analcancer/detailedguide/anal-cancer-risk-factors, 2016 (Accessed Oct 6, 2016).

American Cancer Society: What are the risk factors for breast cancer? http://www.cancer.org/cancer/breastcancer/detailedguide/breast-cancer-risk-factors, 2016 (Accessed Sep 30, 2016).

American Cancer Society: What are the risk factors for cervical cancer? http://www.cancer.org/cancer/cervicalcancer/detailedguide/cervical-cancer-risk-factors, 2016 (Accessed Oct 3, 2016).

American Cancer Society: What are the risk factors for ovarian cancer? http://www.cancer.org/cancer/ovariancancer/detailedguide/ovarian-cancer-risk-factors, 2016 (Accessed Oct 3, 2016).

American Cancer Society: What are the risk factors for penile cancer? http://www.cancer.org/cancer/testicularcancer/detailedguide/testicular-cancer-risk-factors, 2015 (Accessed Oct 5, 2016).

American College of Allergy: Asthma and immunology (ACAAI): latex allergies. Available at www.acaai.org/public/linkpages/latex.htm (Accessed Nov 12, 2016).

American Society Clinical Oncology (ASCO): Risk factors for testicular cancer. http://www.cancer.net/cancer-types/testicular-cancer/risk-factors, 2015 (Accessed Oct 5, 2016).

American Speech Language and Hearing Association: How does your child hear and talk. http://www.asha.org/public/speech/development/01.htm, 2012 (Accessed Mar 8, 2017).

Anandarajah G, Hight E: Spirituality and medical practice: using the HOPE questions as a practical tool for spiritual assessment, *Am Fam Physician* 63(1):81–89, 2001.

Andrews JS: Making the most of the sports physical, *Contemp Pediatr* 14(3):182–205, 1997.

Andriole GL, Crawford ED, Grubb RL III, et al.: for the PLCO Project Team: prostate cancer screening in the randomized prostate, lung, colorectal, and ovarian cancer screening trial: Mortality results after 13 years of follow-up, *JNCI J Natl Cancer Inst* 104(2):125–132, 2012.

Andriole GL, Crawford ED, Grubb RL III, et al.: for the PLCO Project Team: mortality results from a randomized prostate-cancer screening trial, *N Engl J Med* 360:1310–1319, 2009.

Armitage J: Approach to the patient with lymphadenopathy and splenomegaly. In Goldman L, Safer AI, editors: *Goldman's Cecil Medicine*, ed 25, Philadelphia, 2016, Elsevier.

Ashwell M, Gibson S: Waist-to-height ratio as an indicator of 'early health risk': simpler and more predictive than using a 'matrix' based on BMI and waist circumference, *BMJ Open* 6(3):e010159, 2016.

Bamji M, Stone RK, Kaul A, Usmami G, Schachter FF, Wasserman E: Palpable lymph nodes in healthy newborns and infants, *Pediatrics* 78(4):573–575, 1986.

Barkauskas VH, et al.: *Health and physical assessment*, ed 3, St. Louis, 2002, Mosby.

Barlow SE: The expert committee: expert committee recommendations regarding the prevention, assessment, and treatment of child and adolescent overweight and obesity: summary report, *Pediatrics* 120:S164–S192, 2007.

Barrett MJ, Ayub B, Martinez MW: Cardiac auscultation in sports medicine: strategies to improve clinical care, *Curr Sports Med Rep* 11(2):78–84, 2012.

Barton M, Harris RMD: MPH: Does this patient have breast cancer? the screening clinical breast examination: should it be done? How? In Simel DL, Rennie D, editors: *The rational clinical examination: evidence based clinical diagnosis*, McGraw-Hill, 2009, pp 87–98.

Bhattacharyya I, Chehal HK: White lesions, *Otolaryngol Clin North Am* 44:109–131, 2011.

Bochner RE, Gangar M, Belamarich PF: A clinical approach to tonsillitis, tonsillar hypertrophy, and peritonsillar and retropharyngeal abscesses, *Pediatr Rev* 38(2):81–82, 2017.

Cabrera SM, Bright GM, Frane JW, Blethen SL, Lee PA: Age of thelarche and menarche in contemporary US females: a cross-sectional analysis. *J Pediatr Endocrinol Metab* 27(1–2):47–51, 2014, http://dx.doi.org/10.1515/jpem-2013-0286.

Centers for Disease Control and Prevention (CDC): Human papillomavirus (HPV). http://www.cdc.gov/hpv/index.html, 2015 (Accessed Oct 5, 2016).

Centers for Disease Control and Prevention (CDC): Sexually transmitted treatment guidelines: special populations. http://www.cdc.gov/std/tg2015/specialpops.htm, 2015 (Accessed Oct 7, 2016).

Charoenkwan K, Ninunanahaeminda K, Khunamornpong S, et al.: Effects of gel lubricant on cervical cytology, *Acta Cytol* 52(6):654–658, 2008.

Contrera KJ, Wallhagen MI, Mamo SK, Oh ES, Lin FR: Hearing loss health care for older adults, *J Am Board Fam Med* 29(3):394–403, 2016.

Crane BT, Schessel DA, Nedzelski J, et al.: Peripheral vestibular disorders. In Flint PW, Haughey BH, Lund VJ, et al.: *Cummings otolaryngology: head & neck surgery*, ed 5, Philadelphia, 2010, Mosby Elsevier, pp 2328–2345.

Dains J, Baumann L, Scheibel P: *Advanced health assessment and clinical diagnosis in primary care*, ed 5, St. Louis, 2016, Elsevier.

Deepinder F, Braunstein GD: Drug-induced gynecomastia: an evidence-based review, *Expert Opin Drug Saf* 11:779–795, 2012.

DeMuri GP, Wald ER: Acute sinusitis: clinical manifestations and treatment options, *Pediatr Ann* 39(1):34–40, 2010.

Deng T, Jia J, Zhang T, Guo D, Yang L: Cortical versus non-cortical lesions affect expression of Babinski sign, *Neurol Sci* 34(6):855–859, 2013.

Deutsch MB, editor: *Guidelines for the primary care of transgender and gender nonbinary people*, ed 2, UCSF Center of Excellence for Transgender Health, 2016. http://transhealth.ucsf.edu/trans?page=guidelines-home (Accessed Oct 6, 2016).

Dong YH, Lee WY, Basri NA, et al.: The Montreal cognitive assessment is superior to the mini-mental status examination in detecting patients at higher risk of dementia, *Int Psychogeriatr* 24(11):1749–1755, 2012.

Doty RL: Disturbances of smell and taste. In Daroof RB, Fenichel GM, Jankovic J, et al.: *Bradley's neurology in clinical practice*, ed 6, Philadelphia, 2012, Elsevier Saunders, pp 197–204.

Drossman DA: Functional gastrointestinal disorders: history, pathophysiology, clinical features and Rome IV, *Gastroenterology* 150(6):1262–1279, 2016.

Ebell MH: Diagnosis of appendicitis: part 1. History and physical examination, *Am Fam Physician* 15(6):828–830, 2008.

Edge V, Miller M: *Women's health care*, St. Louis, 1994, Mosby.

Elder, J. Enuresis and voiding dysfunction. In Kliegman RM, Stanton BF, St. Geme JW, Schor N, editors: *Nelson textbook of pediatrics*, ed 20, Philadelphia, 2106, Elsevier, pp 2581–2586.e1.

Ewing JA: Screening for Alcoholism using CAGE: cut down, annoyed, guilty, eye opener, *JAMA* 280(2):1904–1905, 1984.

Feldhaus K, et al.: Accuracy of 3 brief screening questions for detecting partner violence in the emergency department, *JAMA* 277(17):1357–1361, 1997.

Fine AM, Nizet V, Mandl KD: Large-scale validation of the Centor and McIsaac scores to predict group a streptococcal pharyngitis, *Arch Intern Med* 172(11):847–852, 104.

Flynn JT, Kaelber DC, Baker-Smith CM, et al.: Clinical practice guideline for screening and management of high blood pressure in children and adolescents, *Pediatrics* 140(3):e20171904, 2017.

Fox GN: Teaching first trimester uterine sizing, *J Fam Pract* 21(5):400–401, 1985.

Garrick JG: Preparticipation orthopedic screening evaluation, *Clin J Sport Med* 14(3):123–126, 2004.

Gilson M, Desai A, Cardoza-Favarato G, et al.: Does gel affect cytology or comfort in the screening papanicolaou smear? *J Am Board Fam Med* 19(4):340–344, 2006.

Goldenring JM, Rosen DS: Getting into adolescent heads: an essential update, *Contemp Pediatr* 21(1):64–90, 2004.

Griffith WF, Stuart GS, Gluck KL, et al.: Vaginal speculum lubrication and its effects on cervical cytology and microbiology, *Contraception* 72(1):60–64, Jul 2005.

Grummer-Strawn LM, Reinold C, Krebs NF: Use of world health organization and CDC growth charts for children aged 0-59 months in the United States, *MMWR Recomm Rep* 1059(RR-9), 2010.

Hamilton BE, Martin JA, Osterman MJK, et al.: Births: final data for 2014. *National Vital Statistics Reports*, vol. 64, no 12. Hyattsville, MD: National Center for Health Statistics, 2015.

Haka-Ikse K, Mian M: Sexuality in children, *Pediatr Rev* 14:10, 1993.

Harer WBJ, Valenzuela G, Lebo D: Lubrication of the vaginal introitus and external speculum had no effect on Papanicolaou smear interpretation/Commentary, *Evid Based Med* 8(3):79, 2003.

Heft MW, Robinson ME: Age differences in suprathreshold sensory function, *Age* 36(1):1–8, 2014.

Herman T, Giladi N, Hausdorff JM: Properties of the 'timed up and go' test: more than meets the eye, *Gerontology* 57:203–210, 2011.

Horner G: Sexual behavior in children. Normal or not? *J Pediatr Health Care* 18(2):57–64, 2004.

Howe LD, Chaturvedi N, Lawlor DA, et al.: Rapid increases in infant adiposity and overweight/obesity in childhood are associated with higher central and brachial blood pressure in early adulthood, *Hypertens* 32(9):1789–1796, 2014.

Huether SE, Rodway G, DeFriez C: Pain, temperature, regulation, sleep, and sensory function. In McCance KL, Huether SE, Brashers VL, et al.: *Pathophysiology: the biologic basis for disease in adults and children*, ed 7, St. Louis, 2014, Elsevier, pp 484–526.

Huether SE: Pain, temperature, regulation, sleep, and sensory function. In McCance KL, Huether SE, Brashers VL, et al.: *Pathophysiology: the biologic basis for disease in adults and children*, ed 6, St. Louis, 2009, Elsevier Mosby, pp 451–524.

International Society Lymphology: The diagnosis and treatment of peripheral lymphedema consensus document of the international society of lymphology. http://www.u.arizona.edu/~witte/ISL.htm, 2013 (Accessed Feb 4, 2017).

Jenny C, Crawford-Jakubiak JE: Committee on Child Abuse and Neglect, American Academy of Pediatrics. The evaluation of children in the primary care setting when sexual abuse is suspected, *Pediatrics* 132(2):e558–e567, 2013. http://pediatrics.aappublications.org/content/pediatrics/132/2/e558.full.pdf (Accessed Feb 7, 2017).

Kalyani RR, Corriere M, Ferrucci L: Age-related and disease-related muscle loss: the effect of diabetes, obesity, and other diseases, *Lancet Diabetes Endocrinol* 2(10):819–829, 2014.

Katsiki N, Mikhailidis DP, Mantzoros CS: Non-alcoholic fatty liver disease and dyslipidemia: an update, *Metabolism* 65(8):1109–1123, 2016.

Kellogg ND: Sexual behaviors in children: evaluation and management, *Am Fam Physician* 82(10):1233–1238, 2010.

Knight JR, et al.: Validity of the CRAFFT substance abuse screening test among adolescent clinic patients, *Arch Pediatr Adolesc Med* 156:607–614, 2002.

Koop CE: *The Surgeon General's letter on child sexual abuse*, Rockville, Md, 1988, U.S. Department of Health and Human Services, Public Health Service.

Köşüş A, Köşüş N, Duran M, et al.: Effect of liquid-based gel application during speculum examination on satisfactory level of smear examination, *Arch Gynecol Obstet* 285:1599–1602, 2012.

Kraft CT, Malhotra S, Boerst A, Thorne MC: Risk indicators for congenital and delayed-onset hearing loss, *Otol Neurotol* 35(10):1839–1843, 2014.

Kulik DM, Uleryk EM, Maguire JL: Does this child have appendicitis? A systematic review of clinical prediction rules for children with acute abdominal pain, *J Clin Epidemiol* 66(1):95–104, 2013.

Landon M, Gabbe SG, Niebyl J, et al.: *Obstetrics: normal and problem pregnancies*, ed 7, Philadelphia, 2017, Elsevier.

Lederle FA, Simel DL: The rational clinical examination. Does this patient have abdominal aortic aneurysm? *JAMA* 281(1):77–82, 1999.

Lederle FA: In the clinic. Abdominal aortic aneurysm, *Ann Intern Med* 150(9), 2009.

LeFevre ML: U.S. Preventive Services Task Force: Screening for abdominal aortic aneurysm: U.S. preventive services task force recommendation statement, *Ann Intern Med* 161(4):281–290, 2014.

Levin SJ, et al.: ETHNIC: a framework for culturally competent clinical practice, *Patient Care* 9(special issue):188, 2000.

Lieberman III JA: BATHE: an approach to the interview process in the primary care setting, *J Clin Psychiatry* 58(Suppl 3):3–6, 1997.

Lin SN, Taylor J, Alperstein S, Hoda R, Holcomb K: Does speculum lubricant affect liquid-based Papanicolaou test adequacy? *Cancer Cytopathology* 122:221–226, 2014.

Lowdermilk DL, Perry SE: *Maternity and women's health care*, ed 8, St. Louis, 2004, Mosby.

Mallants C, Casteels K: Practical approach to childhood masturbation—a review, *Eur J Pediatr* 167(10):1111–1117, 2008.

Marin JR, Alpern ER: Abdominal pain in children, *Emerg Med Clin North Am* 29(2):401–428, ix–x, 2011.

Markowitz LE, Dunne EF, Saraiya M, et al.: Centers for Disease Control and Prevention (CDC): Human papillomavirus vaccination: recommendations of the advisory committee on immunization practices (ACIP), *MMWR Recomm Rep* 63(No. RR-05):1–30, 2014 (Accessed Sep 16, 2016).

Maron BJ, Levine BD, Washington RL, et al.: Eligibility and disqualification recommendations for competitive athletes with cardiovascular abnormalities: Task Force 2: preparticipation screening for cardiovascular disease in competitive athletes: a scientific statement from the American Heart Association and American College of Cardiology, *J Am Coll Cardiol* 66(21):2356–2361, 2015.

Marur S, Forastiere AA: Head and neck squamous cell carcinoma: update on epidemiology, diagnosis, and treatment, *Mayo Clin Proc* 91(3):386–396, 2016.

Maugans TA: The SPIRITual history, *Arch Fam Med* 5(1):11–16, 1996.

McClain N, et al.: Evaluation of sexual abuse in the pediatric patient, *J Pediatr Health Care* 14(3):93–102, 2000.

McCrory P, Meeuwisse W, Aubry M, et al.: Consensus statement on concussion in sport—the 4th International Conference on Concussion in Sport, held in Zurich, November 2012, *Br J Sports Med* 47(5):250–258, 2013.

McShefferty D, et al.: The effect of experience on the sensitivity and specificity of the whispered voice test: a diagnostic accuracy study, *BMJ Open* 3:e002394, 2013.

Merkel S, Voepel-Lewis T, Shayevitz JR, et al.: The FLACC: a behavioral scale for scoring postoperative pain in young children, *Pediatr Nurs* 23(2):293–297, 1997.

Methven L, Allen VJ, Withers CA, Gosney MA: Ageing and taste, *Proc Nutr Soc* 71(4):556–565, 2012.

Milian M, Leiherr AM, Straten G, et al.: The mini-cog versus the mini-mental state examination and the clock drawing test in daily clinical practice: screening value in a German memory clinic, *Int Psychogeriatr* 24(5):766–774, 2012.

Mirabelli MH, Devine MJ, Singh J, Mendoza M: The preparticipation sports evaluation, *Am Fam Physician* 92(5):371–376, 2015.

Miyasaki-Ching CM: *Chasteen's essentials of clinical dental assisting*, ed 5, St. Louis, 1997, Mosby.

Myers ER, Moorman P, Gierisch JM, et al.: Benefits and harms of breast cancer screening: a systematic review, *JAMA* 314(15):1615–1634, 2015.

National Cancer Institute: Genetics of breast and ovarian cancer (PDQ®). https://www.cancer.gov/types/breast/hp/breast-ovarian-genetics-pdq#section/all. Updated February 10, 2017 (Accessed Feb 13, 2017).

National Cancer Institute: Breast Cancer Risk in American Women. https://www.cancer.gov/types/breast/risk-fact-sheet, 2012. Accessed Sept 30, 2016.

National Cancer Institute: Oral cancer prevention PDQ®. http://www.cancer.gov/cancertopics/pdq/prevention/oral/HealthProfessional#Section_121, 2012.

National Heart, Lung, and Blood Institute: Blood pressure tables for children and adolescents from the fourth report on the diagnosis, evaluation, and treatment of high blood pressure in children and adolescents, 2004. Retrieved February 25, 2017. http://www.nhlbi.nih.gov/guidelines/hypertension/child_tbl.htm.

National Institutes of Health: National Heart, Lung, and Blood Institute: The Seventh Report of the Joint National Committee on Prevention, Detection, Evaluation, and Treatment of High Blood Pressure (JNC7), 2004. Retrieved February 25, 2017. http://www.nhlbi.nih.gov/health-pro/guidelines/current/hypertension-jnc-7/complete-report (Accessed Jan 5, 2017).

Nelson HD, Cantor A, Humphrey L, et al.: *Screening for breast cancer: a systematic review to update the 2009 U.S. preventive services task force recommendation.* Evidence Synthesis No. 124. AHRQ Publication No. 14-05201-EF-1. Rockville, MD, 2016, Agency for Healthcare Research and Quality, 2016.

Oeffinger KC, Fontham EH, Etzioni R, et al.: Breast Cancer Screening for Women at Average Risk: 2015 Guideline Update From the American Cancer Society, *JAMA* 314(15):1599–1614, 2015.

Ogden CL, Carroll MD, Fryar CD, et al.: Prevalence of obesity in the United States, 2011-2014, NCHS data brief, 219. https://www.cdc.gov/nchs/data/databriefs/db219.pdf, 2015 (Accessed Feb 6, 2017).

Pawson EG, Petrakis NL: Comparisons of breast pigmentation among women of different racial groups, *Hum Biol* 47:441, 1975.

Petrosky E, Bocchini Jr JA, Hariri S, et al.: Use of 9-valent human papillomavirus (HPV) vaccine: updated HPV vaccination recommendations of the advisory committee on immunization practices, *MMWR 2* 64(11):300–304, 2015.

Phillips-Burkhart K: Why we should screen all patients ages 70 and older for frailty syndrome, *Am Nurse Today* 11(7):7–9, 2016.

Piscascia M, Zangaglia R, Bernini S, Minafra B, Sintoriani E, Pacchetti C: A review of cognitive impairment and differential diagnosis in idiopathic normal pressure hydrocephalus, *Funct Neurol* 30(4):217–228, 2015.

Powell EL, Powell J, Samuel JR, Wilson JA: A review of the pathogenesis of adult peritonsillar abscess: time for a re-evaluation, *J Antimicrob Chemother* 68(9):1941–1950, 2013.

Rademaker J: Hodgkin's and non-Hodgkin's lymphomas, *Radiol Clin North Am* 45(1):69–83, 2007.

Reuter EM, Rehage CV, Vieluf S, Godde B: Touch perception throughout working life: effects of age and expertise, *Exp Brain Res* 216(2):287–297, 2012.

Rossi BV, Ference EH, Zurakowski D, et al.: The clinical presentation and surgical management of adnexal torsion in the pediatric and adolescent population, *J Pediatr Adolesc Gynecol* 25(2):109–113, 2012.

Sanders B, Blackburn TA, Bourcher B: Preparticipation screening—the sports physical therapy perspective, *Int J Sports Phys Ther* 8(2):180–193, 2013.

Schröder FH, Hugosson J, Roobol M, et al.: for the ERSPC Investigators: screening and prostate-cancer mortality in a randomized European study, *N Engl J Med* 360:1320–1328, 2009.

Schröder FH, Hugosson J, Roobol MJ, et al.: Prostate-cancer mortality at 11 years of follow-up, *N Engl J Med* 366:981–990, 2012.

Sheikh JL, Yesavage JA: Geriatric depression scale: recent evidence and development of a shorter version, *Clin Gerontol* 5:165–172, 1986.

Sherin KM, et al.: HITS: a short domestic violence screening tool for use in a family practice setting, *Fam Med* 30(7):508–512, 1998.

Silk H: Diseases of the mouth, *Prim Care* 41(1):75–90, 2014.

Simel DL: Update: ascites. In Simel DL, Rennie D, editors: *The rational clinical examination evidence-based clinical diagnosis*, New York, 2009, McGraw Hill.

Simel DL, Williams JW: Update: sinusitis. In Simel DL, Rennie D, editors: *The rational clinical examination: evidence-based clinical diagnosis*, New York, 2009, McGraw Hill Medical, pp 601–602.

Sokol RJ, et al.: TACE questions: practical prenatal detection of risk-drinking, *Am J Obstet Gyencol* 260(4):863–868, 1989.

Stuart MR, Lieberman JA: The fifteen minute hour. In *Applied psychotherapy for the primary care physician*, ed 2, Westport, CT and London, 1993, Praeger.

Studdiford J, Lamb K, Horvath K, et al.: Development of unilateral cervical and supraclavicular lymphadenopathy after human papillomavirus vaccination, *Pharmacotherapy* 28(9):1194–1197, 2008.

Tan HL, Kheirandish-Gozal L, Abel F, Gozal D: Craniofacial syndromes and sleep-related breathing disorders, *Sleep Med Rev* 27:74–88, 2016.

Thompson JM, McFarland GK, Hirsch JE, Taylor SM: *Clinical nursing*, ed 4, St. Louis, 1997, Mosby.

Tinetti ME: Performance-oriented assessment of mobility problems in elderly patients, *J Am Geriatr Soc* 34(2):119–126, 1986.

Uçar A, Saka N, Baş F, Bundak R, Günöz H, Darendeliler F: Is premature thelarche in the first two years of life transient? *J Clin Res Pediatr Endocrinol* 4(3):140–145, 2012.

U.S. Preventive Services Task Force (USPSTF): *Final recommendation statement: colorectal cancer screening*, Rockville, MD, 2016, U.S. Dept. of Health & Human Services, Agency for Healthcare Research and Quality.

U.S. Preventive Services Task Force (USPSTF).: *Final Evidence Summary: Hearing Loss in Older Adults: Screening*. August 2012. https://www.uspreventiveservicestaskforce.org/Page/Document/final-evidence-summary29/hearing-loss-in-older-adults-screening, (Accessed March 18, 2017).

U.S. Preventive Services Task Force (USPSTF). Abdominal Aortic Aneurysm: Screening. June 2014. http://www.uspreventiveservicestaskforce.org/Page/Document/UpdateSummaryFinal/abdominal-aortic-aneurysm-screening (Accessed March 18, 2017).

U.S. Preventive Services Task Force (USPSTF): *Final update summary: abdominal*, July 2015. http://www.uspreventiveservicestaskforce.org/Page/Document/UpdateSummaryFinal/abdominal-aortic-aneurysm-screening (Accessed March 18, 2017).

US Preventive Services Task Force: Breast cancer: screening. https://www.uspreventiveservicestaskforce.org/Page/Document/UpdateSummaryFinal/breast-cancer-screening1?ds=1&s=breast, 2016 (Accessed Feb 13, 2017).

U.S. Preventive Services Task Force. Final Recommendation Statement Cervical Cancer: *Screening*, https://www.uspreventiveservicestaskforce.org/Page/Document/RecommendationStatementFinal/cervical-cancer-screening#rationale, 2012. (Accessed July 20, 2017).

US Preventive Services Task Force: Prostate cancer: screening. Final recommendation statement. https://www.uspreventiveservicestaskforce.org/Page/Document/RecommendationStatementFinal/prostate-cancer-screening, 2012 (Accessed Oct 6, 2016).

Van Laer L, Dietz H, Loeys B: Loeys-Dietz Syndrome, *Adv Exp Med Biol* 802:95–105, 2014.

Veloso FT: Clinical predictors of Crohn's disease course, *Eur J Gastroenterol Hepatol* 28:1122–1125, 2016.

Vieira AR: Unravelling human cleft lip and palate research, *J Dent Res* 87(2):119–125, 2008.

Waghdhare S, Kalantri A, Joshi R, Kalantri S: Accuracy of physical signs for detecting meningitis: a hospital-based diagnostic accuracy study, *Clin Neurol Neurosurg* 112(9):752–757, 2010.

Wagner J: Update: appendicitis, adult. In Simel DL, Rennie D, editors: *The rational clinical examination evidence-based clinical diagnosis*, New York, 2009, McGraw Hill.

Warden V, Hurley AC, Volicer L: Development and psychometric evaluation of the pain assessment in advanced dementia (PAINAD) scale, *J Am Med Dir Assoc* 4:9–15, 2003.

Watson JC, Dyck JB: Peripheral neuropathy: a practical guide for diagnosis and symptom management, *Mayo Clin Proc* 90(7):940–951, 2015.

Wilson SF, Giddens JF: *Health assessment for nursing practice*, ed 4, St. Louis, 2009, Mosby.

Womack J: Give your sports physicals a performance boost, *J Fam Pract* 59(8):437–444, 2010.

Won AC, Ethell A: Spontaneous splenic rupture resulted from infectious mononucleosis, *Int J Surg Case Rep* 3(3):97–99, 2012.

Wren T: Penile and testicular disorders, *Nurs Clin North Am* 39:319, 2004.

Zardawi IM, Catterall N, Duncan J, Sullivan J, Warwick L: Effects of lubricant gel on conventional and liquid-based cervical smears [letter], *Acta Cytol* 47(4):704–705, 2003.

Quick Reference to Special Histories

CAGE Questionnaire: A Framework for Detecting Alcoholism

The CAGE questionnaire was developed in 1984 by Dr. John Ewing, and it includes
four interview questions designed to help diagnose alcoholism. The acronym
"CAGE" helps practitioners quickly recall the main concepts of the four questions
(**C**utting down, **A**nnoyance by criticism, **G**uilty feeling, **E**ye-openers).

Probing questions may be asked as follow-up questions to the CAGE questionnaire.
Many online resources list the complete questionnaire (e.g., http://addictionsand
recovery.org/addiction-self-test.htm). The exact wording of the CAGE Questionnaire can be found in Ewing JA: Screening for Alcoholism using CAGE: cut down,
annoyed, guilty, eye opener, *JAMA* 280(2): 1904-1905, 1984.

TACE Questionnaire: A Framework for Prenatal Detection of Risk Drinking

MNEMONIC	QUESTIONS
T: Take	How many drinks does it take to make you feel high? (More than two drinks suggests a tolerance to alcohol that is a red flag.) How many when you first started drinking? When was that? Which do you prefer: beer, wine, or liquor?
A: Annoyed	Have people annoyed you by criticizing your drinking?
C: Cut down	Have you felt you ought to cut down on your drinking?
E: Eye-opener	Have you ever had an eye-opener drink first thing in the morning to steady your nerves or get rid of a hangover?

A positive answer to **T** alone or to two of **A, C,** or **E** may signal a alcohol problem
with a high degree of probability, and positive answers to all four, signal this with
great certainty.

From Sokol RJ, et al: TACE questions: practical prenatal detection of risk-drinking, *Am J Obstet Gynecol*
260(4):863–868, 1989.

The CRAFFT Questionnaire: A Framework for Detecting Recreational Substance Use Disorders in Adolescents

The CRAFFT questionnaire was developed in 2002 as a screening tool for alcohol and substance abuse in adolescents. The CRAFFT acronym helps practitioners remember the main concepts of the six questions: **C**ar, **R**elax, **A**lone, **F**orget, **F**riends, **T**rouble.

The exact wording of the CRAFFT questions can be found here: Knight JR et al., Validity of the CRAFFT Substance Abuse Screening Test Among Adolescent Clinic Patients. *Arch Pediatr Adolesc Med* 156:607-614, 2002 (available online at http://archpedi.jamanetwork.com/article.aspx?articleid=203511).

Domestic Violence: Three Questions as a Brief Screening Instrument

1. Have you been hit, kicked, punched, or otherwise hurt by someone within the past year?
2. Do you feel safe in your current relationship?
3. Is a partner from a previous relationship making you feel unsafe now?

A positive response to any one of these three questions constitutes a positive screen for partner violence.

The first question, which addresses physical violence, has been validated in studies as an accurate measure of 1-year prevalence rates.

The last two questions evaluate the perception of safety and estimate the short-term risk of further violence and the need for counseling, but reliability and validity evaluations have not yet been established.

From MacMillan HL, Wathen CN, Jamieson E, Boyle M, McNutt L, Worster A, Lent B, Webb M, McMaster Violence Against Women Research Group FT. Approaches to Screening for Intimate Partner Violence in Health Care Settings: A Randomized Trial. *JAMA.* 2006;296(5):530-536. http://dx.doi.org/10.1001/jama.296.5.530.

Brief Screening Tool for Domestic Violence: HITS

Verbal abuse is as intense a problem as physical violence. **HITS** stands for **H**urt, **I**nsult, **T**hreaten, or **S**cream. The wording of the question is, "In the last year, how often did your partner:

Hurt you physically?"
Insult or talk down to you?"
Threaten you with physical harm?"
Scream or curse at you?"

BATHE Questionnaire: A Framework for Understanding the Patient in the Context of His or Her Total Life Situation

MNEMONIC	QUESTIONS
B: Background	What is going on in your life? What is going on right now? Has anything changed recently?
A: Affect	How do you feel about that? What is your mood?
T: Trouble	What about the situation troubles you most? What worries or concerns you?
H: Handling	How are you handling that? How are you coping?
E: Empathy	That must be very difficult for you. I can understand that you would feel that way.

The fifteen minute hour: applied psychotherapy for the primary care physician by Lieberman, Joseph A., III; Stuart, Marian R. Reproduced with permission of Greenwood Publishing Group, Incorporated in the format Republish in a book via Copyright Clearance Center.

FICA Questionnaire: A Framework for Spiritual Assessment

MNEMONIC	QUESTIONS
F: Faith, Belief, Meaning	What is your spiritual or religious heritage? Is the Bible, the Quran, or similar writings important to you? Do these beliefs help you cope with stress?
I: Importance and Influence	How have these beliefs influenced how you handle stress? To what extent?
C: Community	Do you belong to a formal spiritual or religious community? Does this community support you? In what way? Is there anyone there with whom you would like to talk?
A: Address/Action in Care	How do your religious beliefs affect your healthcare decisions (e.g., choice of birth control)? How would you like me to support you in this regard when your health is involved?

Adapted from Puchalski, C; Romer, Al. Taking a Spiritual History Allows Clinicians to Understand Patients More Fully. *J Palliat Med.* 3, 1, 129, 2000. ISSN: 10966218.

ETHNIC Questionnaire: A Framework for Culturally Competent Clinical Practice

MNEMONIC	QUESTIONS
E: Explanation	Why do you think you have these symptoms? What do friends, family, and others say? Do you know others with this problem? Have you seen it on TV, heard about it on the radio, or read about it in the newspaper?
T: Treatment	Do you take any treatments, medicines, or home remedies to treat the illness or to stay healthy? What kinds of treatment are you seeking from me?
H: Healers	Have you sought advice from friends, alternative folk healers, or other nondoctors?
N: Negotiate	Negotiate mutually acceptable options; incorporate patient's beliefs. Ask what results patient hopes to achieve from intervention.
I: Intervention	Determine an intervention with your patient. May include incorporation of alternative treatments, spirituality, healers, or other cultural practices (e.g., foods to be eaten or avoided).
C: Collaborate	Collaborate with the patient, family, health team members, healers, and community resources.

Modified from Levin SJ, et al: ETHNIC: A framework for culturally competent clinical practice, *Patient Care* 9(special issue):188, 2000.

The HEEADSSS Psychosocial Interview for Adolescents (Essential Questions)

MNEMONIC	QUESTIONS
H: Home	Who lives with you? Where do you live? Do you have your own room? What are relationships like at home? To whom are you closest at home? To whom can you talk at home? Is there anyone new at home? Has someone left recently? Have you moved recently? Have you ever had to live away from home? (Why?)

The HEEADSSS Psychosocial Interview for Adolescents (Essential Questions)—cont'd

MNEMONIC	QUESTIONS
E: Education and employment	What are your favorite subjects at school? Your least favorite subjects? How are your grades? Any recent changes? Any dramatic changes in the past? Have you changed schools in the past few years? What are your future education/employment plans/goals? Are you working? Where? How much?
E: Eating	What do you like and not like about your body? Have there been any recent changes in your weight? Have you dieted in the last year? How? How often? Have you done anything else to try to manage your weight? How much exercise do you get in an average day? Week? What do you think would be a healthy diet? How does that compare to your current eating patterns?
A: Activities	What do you and your friends do for fun? (With whom, where, and when?) What do you and your family do for fun? (With whom, where, and when?) Do you participate in any sports or other activities? Do you regularly attend a church group, club, or other organized activity?
D: Drugs	Do you and your friends use tobacco? Alcohol? Other drugs? Does anyone in your family use tobacco? Alcohol? Other drugs? Do you use tobacco? Alcohol? Other drugs? Is there any history of alcohol or drug problems in your family? Does anyone at home use tobacco?
S: Sexuality	Have you ever been in a romantic relationship? Tell me about the people that you've dated. OR Tell me about your sex life. Have any of your relationships ever been sexual relationships? Are your sexual activities enjoyable? What does the term "safer sex" mean to you?
S: Suicide and depression	Do you feel sad or down more than usual? Do you feel yourself crying more than usual? Are you "bored" all the time? Are you having trouble getting to sleep? Have you thought a lot about hurting yourself or someone else?

The HEEADSSS Psychosocial Interview for Adolescents (Essential Questions)—cont'd

MNEMONIC	QUESTIONS
S: Safety (savagery)	Have you ever been seriously injured? (How?) How about anyone else you know? Do you always wear a seatbelt in the car? Have you ever ridden with a driver who was drunk or high? When? How often? Do you use safety equipment for sports and/or other physical activities (e.g., helmets for biking or skateboarding)? Is there any violence at your school? In your neighborhood? Among your friends? Have you ever been physically or sexually abused? Have you ever been raped, on a date or at any other time? (if not asked previously)

Index

Note: Page numbers followed by *f* indicate figures; *t*, tables; *b*, boxes.

INDEX

INDEX

INDEX

INDEX

CDC and WHO Growth Charts

Reference these growth charts at http://www.cdc.gov/growthcharts/who_charts.htm

Who Growth Charts

Birth to 24 Months

Boys Length-for-Age Percentiles and Weight-for-Age Percentiles

Boys Weight-for-Length Percentiles and Head Circumference-for-Age Percentiles

Girls Length-for-Age Percentiles and Weight-for-Age Percentiles

Girls Weight-for-Length Percentiles and Head Circumference-for-Age Percentiles

CDC Growth Charts

Children and Adolescents 2 to 20 Years (5th-95th Percentile)

Boys Stature-for-Age and Weight-for-Age

Boys BMI-for-Age

Girls Stature-for-age and Weight-for-Age

Girls BMI-for-Age

Optional Charts (5th-95th Percentile)

Boys Weight-for-Stature

Girls Weight-for-Stature